Living with risk

Mental health service user involvement in risk assessment and management

Joan Langan and Vivien Lindow

First published in Great Britain in April 2004 by

The Policy Press
Fourth Floor, Beacon House
Queen's Road
Bristol BS8 1QU
UK

Tel no +44 (0)117 331 4054
Fax no +44 (0)117 331 4093
E-mail tpp-info@bristol.ac.uk
www.policypress.org.uk

© Joseph Rowntree Foundation/The Policy Press 2004

Published for the Joseph Rowntree Foundation by The Policy Press

ISBN 1 86134 596 8

British Library Cataloguing in Publication Data
A catalogue record for this report is available from the British Library.

Library of Congress Cataloging-in-Publication Data
A catalog record for this report has been requested.

Joan Langan is a Lecturer in the School for Policy Studies, University of Bristol and **Vivien Lindow** is a freelance psychologist working from the perspective of a former mental health service user.

The **Joseph Rowntree Foundation** has supported this project as part of its programme of research and innovative development projects, which it hopes will be of value to policy makers, practitioners and service users. The facts presented and views expressed in this report are, however, those of the authors and not necessarily those of the Foundation.

Cover design by Qube Design Associates, Bristol
Printed in Great Britain by Hobbs the Printers Ltd, Southampton

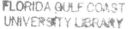

Contents

Acknowledgements

We would like to thank the service users who were willing to discuss with us the difficult and sensitive area of risk, and in particular risk to other people. We also want to thank the relatives, friends and professionals who were willing to discuss this complex area. Thanks are also due to Catherine Anglim and Jill Redmayne for their assistance with interviewing and data inputting and to Tara Mistry and Azra Sangster who carried out some of the interviews. We are also grateful for the valuable input of John Boardman and Frank Keating who acted as consultants and to the Research Advisory Group who shared their expertise with us.

Finally, given the difficult personal circumstances that we both experienced during the research period, we are grateful for the unfailing support of the Joseph Rowntree Foundation.

Glossary

The study took place in England and the following information about law and policy is correct for that country.

Actuarial prediction

This means prediction based on what research suggests are significant risk factors, for example age, gender and previous history of violence.

Care Programme Approach (CPA)

This is the bedrock of mental health policy and practice and applies to everyone who is accepted as a client of specialist mental health services. Every psychiatric in-patient should receive a CPA before being discharged. The CPA has four elements:

- systematic assessment of the person's health and social care needs;
- the development of a care plan to meet those assessed needs;
- a named keyworker to be the main point of contact between the service user and professionals delivering the care plan;
- regular review and monitoring of the care plan.

Section 117 of the 1983 Mental Health Act

Section 117 imposes a duty on health trusts and social services departments, in conjunction with relevant voluntary agencies, to provide aftercare services for people subject to sections 3, 37, 47 and 48 of the Act. There is no obligation on the person concerned to accept the services.

Under Section

A person under section is subject to powers of compulsory detention under the 1983 Mental Health Act.

Supervised discharge

Via the 1995 Mental Health (Patients in the Community) Act, supervised discharge (or 'aftercare under supervision') imposes additional requirements on a person who is subject to section 117 of the 1983 Mental Health Act where s/he is

- suffering from one of the four categories of mental disorder defined in S1(2) of the Act;

and

- there would be a substantial risk of serious harm to the health and safety of the patient, or the safety of other persons, or of the person being seriously exploited, if the patient did not receive after-care services under section 117 of the Act;

and

- that supervision is likely to help ensure that the patient receives those services. (LAC [96]8)

The person can be required to live at a specified place and attend for medical treatment, occupation or education, as well as make themselves available to be seen by their nominated supervisor, any doctor, approved social worker (the social worker who has powers under the 1983 Mental Health Act, including to make the application for compulsory admission or detention) or any other person authorised by the supervisor.

Supervision register

The aim is to ensure that people who may be a serious risk to themselves or other people do not disengage from services. The register holds information about the person's status under the Mental Health Act, the risk behaviours, details of the care plan and which professionals are involved. The government (DoH, 1999a) has recommended that they no longer be used.

Introduction

This research is about the involvement in risk assessment and management of those mental health service users considered by professionals to pose a potential risk to other people. The research was carried out because of concerns that the voices of such service users were not being heard in research, policy or practice. Our overall aim is to produce recommendations for good practice that enable the expertise of this largely hidden group to be included in the planning and provision of effective services. This chapter outlines the aims and objectives of the research and then describes the context of increasing concern about dangerousness within which it took place, a fact noted by the following service user, who also identified more salient risk factors than mental state, namely age and gender:

"But, again, from the kind of general voice of users who say 'Well, actually, most of us find that a little bit kind of strong to somehow say because one's had mental health problems, you're immediately at risk to the public'.... And so, you know, to put it in context, all those lads out on Saturday nights supporting England are probably much more of a risk to the general public than I am with my mental health difficulties."

The lack of research exploring the views of service users defined as a risk to others is also highlighted in this chapter. Finally, we describe details of the criteria developed to find a sample of service users and details of how we wrote up the research to preserve anonymity and confidentiality.

Project aims and objectives

The project's aims and objectives are as follows:

- to provide information about the extent to which people defined as a risk to others are being involved in the assessment and management of any risk;
- to explore the extent to which service users, professionals and families or close friends (where appropriate) agree about the level and nature of any risk and its management;
- to explore how helpful service users find the support they receive in terms of managing risk;
- to provide information about how risk is assessed and managed within community care services;
- to produce guidelines informed by service users about the management of risk to others among mental health service users living in the community.

We hope that the research will be useful to a number of different audiences in that it will:

- provide an opportunity for people who become a risk to others during an episode of mental distress to speak about their experiences and about what is helpful to them in terms of managing risk;
- encourage mental health service user groups to support more members of this minority group;
- provide information on providing services to people defined as a risk to others which are acceptable to them and which protect them from harming others;
- contribute to national mental health policy;
- be valuable to commissioners and providers of local services in terms of how risk assessment and management might be improved by involving service users.

Policy and research background

Policy

One of the consequences of the reduction in psychiatric hospital beds and the expansion of services in the community since the early 1990s is media and public alarm about the presence of mental health service users in the community.

The tendency towards greater control over people diagnosed as mentally ill appears to be motivated by public concern, fed by some sections of the media, rather than evidence about the best way to ensure public safety. For example, Parker and McCulloch's (1999) examination of homicide enquiries found that, in order of importance, poor risk management, communication problems, inadequate care planning, lack of inter-agency working, administrative and procedural failures, lack of suitable accommodation, poor resources and substance misuse were more significant factors than what is commonly seen as the reason for the presence of risk – non-compliance with medication.

What is striking, when looking back over the past decade of mental health policy, is the ever-increasing focus on risk, and particularly risk to other people. There was no mention of risk at all in the circular introducing the Care Programme Approach (CPA) within England (DoH, 1990). Since then, mental health service users have become increasingly defined in terms of the risk that they are seen as presenting rather than in terms of their needs and rights, despite consistent research evidence (Steadman et al, 1998; Langan, 1999) that people defined as mentally ill make either no or minimal contributions to violence. As mental health policy has moved further in the direction of controlling individuals considered to be a risk to others, assessing and managing risk has also become a key requirement for mental health professionals. In 1994 came the first mention of the requirement on professionals to conduct risk assessments and develop a risk management plan for people being discharged from hospital (DoH, 1994). British policy or guidance establishes that service users should be involved in the process of risk assessment and management (DoH, 1999a; Scottish Executive, 2000). However, there is no real detail on how to actually do this other than

that the assessment should be holistic and consider the need for positive risk taking (DoH, 1999a).

Yet defensive practice is the more likely outcome. Although most government guidance stresses that the majority of people with mental health problems present no risk to other people, this is invariably after a discussion of the small minority who may be. Government pronouncements have also been extremely unhelpful in associating mental health problems with dangerousness, for example, "the tragic toll of homicides" (DoH, 2000, p 1). This is despite research (Taylor and Gunn, 1999) showing that, although there has been a fivefold increase in homicides over the period 1957-99, the figures for people defined as mentally ill show a decrease of 3% per annum. We would not wish to deny, however, that anyone who is killed or injured by a person diagnosed as mentally ill is deeply regrettable as well as tragic. Welsh Office policy guidance (National Assembly for Wales, 2001, p 22) is more measured in its appraisal of risk, saying:

> It is important that the legitimate and desirable aim of reducing public anxiety does not drive policy on mental health services inappropriately. (p 22)

The Draft Mental Health Bill for England and Wales (DoH, 2002a) continues the government's focus on coercion and concordance without giving service users a right to services that would be much more effective in terms of reducing rare dangers. Paradoxically, the government is encouraging service user involvement and seeking to counter the stigma experienced by people with a diagnosis of mental illness, a stigma exacerbated by their own focus on the small minority of people who are a risk to others when experiencing psychosis. Indeed, the Health Select Committee (2000, section 39, website) stated:

> We feel that it is both misleading and unhelpful to state the policy of community care has failed as the government has done on numerous occasions.

Research

While a considerable body of work exists about the support that mental health service users want for themselves (Faulkner and Layzell, 2000; Keating et al, 2002), little, if any, research has been carried out about the issues that people defined as a risk to others believe are important. The psychiatric literature concentrates on global features of the person's mental state, for example, seeking to develop valid instruments to measure the relationship of delusions or anger to subsequent violence. While useful, this provides little information at the individual level (Scottish Executive 2000; Petch, 2001). Sayce (1995) asserts the urgency of disseminating good practice in working with users to identify triggers to anger. She also states that service users' experience of being violent, their perceptions of causes, triggers and help required, as well as their ability to predict violence, are under-researched. Indeed, one of the few research studies in this area (Estroff and Zimmer, 1994) found that people who were violent were often involved in family relationships characterised by hostility and tension. Such research shows that we need to consider the context within which violence takes place and not necessarily assume that the problem lies within the individual or that it is necessarily due to 'mental illness'.

What is missing from the debate, and the proposed solutions, is the voice of individuals who are seen to pose a risk to others. Robinson's[1] (1997) autobiography makes it clear that some service users are unable to accept that they can be dangerous. However, many service users are aware of the risks that they can pose to other people and want help to reduce those risks (Campbell and Lindow, 1997).

The situation of service users from minority ethnic communities is of particular concern. There is clear statistical evidence of over-diagnosing of schizophrenia, involuntary admission and referral to psychiatric services from the courts among some minority groups (Fernando, 1995). Institutional racism throughout the mental health system, including within the forensic services, is a matter of record (Browne, 1997; Fernando et al, 1998). Again,

within the research literature there is some evidence about what service users themselves expect (Wilson and Francis, 1997), but little in relation to risk assessment and management.

How professionals manage the dilemmas involved in balancing protection and autonomy is another under-researched area. One study (Emerson and Pollner, 1975) found that mental health professionals using compulsory powers in situations where they felt there was little alternative, described their work as 'shit-work' and did not subject this work to critical scrutiny.

In conclusion, the continued focus on risk means that there is a real danger that people defined as a risk to others will increasingly be seen as an 'underclass' in society (Sayce, 1995) and that they will not be properly involved in decisions about their own lives, or have a say over the support given to them. The current political, cultural and policy climate also means that they risk further exclusion and marginalisation.

The research

The focus of this research is people being discharged from in-patient treatment and moving into the community. The research design was in-depth interviews with service users at the point of hospital discharge (Phase 1) and six months later (Phase 2). We planned to carry out in-depth interviews with 20 services users but, in the event, received consent from 17 service users. Of these, two service users were women and four service users were from minority ethnic groups. With the service user's consent we also interviewed up to three mental health professionals at each interview point, as well as a relative or friend. Professionals interviewed included: psychiatrists, community psychiatric nurses, social workers, psychologists, housing workers and daycare staff. The total number of interviews carried out was 129.

The Appendix contains more information about the research design, the difficulties we encountered in doing this research, as well as details of those interviewed.

---

[1] Andrew Robinson killed an occupational therapist while an in-patient in a psychiatric hospital.

Criteria for referral to the project

Eight hospital-based consultant psychiatrists (including three locum consultants) and their teams cooperated with our research. We asked them to refer people aged between 18-65 living within a set geographical area whom they considered to pose a possible risk to others, with the criteria for risk being:

- currently or previously subject to supervised discharge;
- currently or previously placed on a supervision register;
- violent behaviour;
- physical, sexual or emotional abuse of children;
- domestic violence;
- violence on the ward;
- making threats about other people that causes serious concern.

These criteria were developed after meetings with consultant psychiatrists to plan the research.

Service users not included in the research

When liaising with consultant psychiatrists about who could be asked to participate in the research, it became clear that some service users could not be asked because they did not know that they were considered to pose a potential risk to other people. This is an important finding and is discussed in more detail in Chapter 4.

Preserving confidentiality

We promised anonymity and confidentiality to everyone interviewed. This was particularly important given the sensitivity of the subject area and the impact on service users if it was known that they were considered to pose a potential risk to other people. We ensured anonymity and confidentiality by:

- not revealing where the research took place;
- assigning male gender to all service users, except where the discussion is specific to women. Our decision was based on the premise that some risk behaviour to others is more significant or threatening when carried out by a man;

- not presenting any material on a 'case study' basis since this would make service users more easily identifiable;
- occasionally changing information that does not alter the research findings but which might allow someone to be identified;
- randomly assigning gender to professionals, relatives and friends.

The risks

In this chapter we discuss accounts of:

- risk behaviour to others;
- risk behaviour to self;
- risks or harm that people experienced from others.

We then discuss the significance of these circumstances as triggers to service users' mental health deteriorating. However, information about the behaviour of the service users in the study comes with the following caution. For some service users, there were discrepancies in accounts, not only between service users and others, but also between professionals, as well as conflicting or inaccurate information held on case files. Where everyone involved agreed about risk, it is possible to be more confident that the accounts of behaviour were accurate, but certainty about the extent and type of risk was impossible for all the service users in this study.

Risk to others

The risk behaviour of people in the study is described as including: assaults; physical aggression; serious verbal threats, including to kill others such as their own children, staff or other residents; verbal aggression; and inappropriate sexual behaviour towards women. Some people had attacked or threatened others with weapons, in some cases actually producing a weapon and in other cases saying that they wanted to use a weapon, such as a knife. We also use the term 'incidental harm' to describe actions such as reckless pedestrian behaviour in fast traffic, dangerous driving, fire-setting or other behaviour designed to destroy perceived enemy action. While some of these behaviours had occurred in the past, all the service users were

seen by professionals as presenting a potential risk to others at or during their period of hospitalisation. However, in a few cases risk to self was considered more significant.

Sometimes staff were unclear whether an assault or threat was a direct result of psychosis or completely unrelated. For example, one man, who agreed that he was a risk to other people and himself when experiencing psychosis, had been provoked into many fights with other men, sometimes due to racist abuse. His response of carrying a weapon at times to protect himself may not be that unusual among young men living in inner cities. However, this defensive action would certainly exacerbate risk if he became out of control when experiencing psychosis. Another service user was described by a professional in the following terms:

"And, you know, it's not purely a mental health issue, that side of things for X. Let's say in a neighbourhood where violence is quite high and certainly he's done jobs where that kind of male, perhaps, behaviour is more acceptable or deemed more acceptable.... Certainly, you know, alcohol is an on-going issue with X, which is a disinhibiting factor that ups the risks again, I suppose."

This comment shows the importance of understanding base rates, that is, the normal frequency of violence in a particular population. For example, a person in a rural area is less likely to act in a violent manner than someone in an urban area, even if they have known risk factors for violence. Indeed, Steadman et al (1998) found that when people defined as mentally ill and discharged into the community were compared with demographically similar control subjects, levels of violence were the same.

While public alarm has been focused by the media on 'stranger danger', that is, random attacks on strangers by people who have used mental health services, those most at risk from the people we met were family members, mental health staff and fellow patients and residents. While the number of service users in this study is small, this finding is in line with other research (Appleby, 2001) about who is most likely to be at risk from the minority of service users who can be a danger to others.

Involvement with the criminal justice system

Six people had been in prison with convictions for assault, actual bodily harm, grievous bodily harm (stabbing), robbery or threatening behaviour. There had also been police involvement in some of the incidents leading up to admission to hospital.

Legal status on admission and whether admission was necessary

We had assumed that everyone in the study would have been sectioned due to concerns about risk to others and although this was the case for the majority, a few were informal patients. All the professionals and relatives or friends thought that hospital admission had been necessary. Service users' views ranged from requesting admission through to ambivalence or accepting hospital as a necessary evil in lieu of other ways of dealing with their difficulties. A small number actively resisted admission. Nine service users had not wanted to be admitted to hospital although two said that that they realised, with hindsight, that it had been necessary. Another two service users were more ambivalent, with one saying that "hospital brings me down" but he could not think of any alternative and the other saying that he had not wanted to go into hospital or be sectioned but he felt that treatment had been helpful. Staff said that another two service users had mentioned the benefit of feeling safe in hospital although not wishing to be there. At the second interview, four people

were still under section (although not necessarily in hospital) either because they did not agree that they needed treatment, did not want it in a hospital setting or wanted to return home. By the second interview, one person was spending more time in hospital than at home and another five service users were admitted between the two interviews, although in one case this was due to physical health problems. They had contrasting views about the benefits of readmission:

"If I become unwell or I'm unstable for a while, I can always come in for a week or two, which is good really."

"Well, I'm not going to go into hospital again anyway, 'cos if I did I'd run away. I'd just hitch a ride to [town] and disappear."

Suicide, self-harm and neglect

Research reviewed by Langan (1999) consistently shows that people with a diagnosis of mental illness are much more likely to be at risk from self-harm or suicide than be a risk to other people. As one service user said:

"And I think it's inevitable, if you've got a serious mental illness, that suicide is a big option because why go on with this horrible life? ... I think if you speak to most people who've had a mental illness, suicide has been a big part of their thinking because it's a disastrous illness to have. It not only takes your dignity away, it takes your mind away and you become isolated, and you're scared, and your life's ruined. It's a terrible thing to have."

Ten people had made suicide attempts, in four cases some considerable time previously and five other people had fears or thoughts of suicide. We arrived at these figures by pooling information from workers, service users, relatives and friends since it was not always the case that everyone working with a particular service user mentioned a suicide attempt. Risk to self was seen as an equally, if not more, important reason for admission for three service users. However, people did not fit into clear categories of either being a suicide risk or not. At times, some service users were seen as more of a risk to themselves than to others and views about seriousness of risk also varied over time. Of those people who had made suicide attempts, one person continued to be actively suicidal by the second interview and as a result was spending more time in hospital than at home. A few service users were coping with voices telling them to kill themselves and in some cases staff were actively working with them to try and reduce the chances that they might act on them.

Self-harm, for example in the form of self-cutting or self-burning, was also an issue for nine service users, with six having engaged in this type of behaviour currently or in the recent past. Six people were seen as vulnerable to danger from others within their community. This ranged from mixing with unsavoury characters in order to acquire illicit drugs or because, in one case, the service user was giving away money to children in the neighbourhood. Four people had walked into traffic recklessly or lain down in front of approaching traffic and this had put themselves and others at risk.

Other harms

Racism

The four service users from minority ethnic groups had all experienced racism, with one saying:

> "Racism is involved in *everything* I've been through."

Three of these service users had been attacked or abused, in two cases recently, because of their ethnic background. One service user said that he had been attacked in prison three times, attacked by a neighbour as well as by strangers in the street. One racial attack had happened while on hospital leave but no staff mentioned supporting him with the consequences, including to his mental health, of being beaten up. Another service user had been attacked while in hospital but professional accounts did not mention racism and it was not clear whether the possibility of racism being involved was discussed. The third service user was described by a worker as having been racially abused by another patient. He had retaliated aggressively and had ended up first in prison and then in a secure psychiatric facility.

One service user had been housed in an area characterised by tension between different minority ethnic groups and both he and a relative had been attacked and threatened. The only drop-in centre was primarily for members of the same minority ethnic group that had attacked him and which he did not want to attend.

Other attacks

Three white service users had also been attacked or threatened with violence and a fourth moved in drug circles where he had been threatened and where he was likely to be attacked. A fifth service user was considered to be vulnerable to getting into dangerous situations and being beaten. Four service users were seen as behaving in ways that increased the risk that they would be attacked by others - for example, preaching to people or being aggressive or confrontational to others when experiencing psychosis.

Neglect

Five service users were also considered by friends, relatives or workers to neglect themselves when experiencing psychosis, for example failing to eat or look after themselves or their property before admission. Service users did not necessarily agree with these views.

Trauma

Several people had experienced traumatic childhoods either due to physical or sexual abuse or through fleeing a war-torn country, being in care, seeing a relative murdered or through having difficult family relationships. The following quotation from a professional refers to a service user whose mental health difficulties were seen as originating from his earlier sexual abuse:

> "So X shows all the typical pattern of difficulties and symptoms that are now well recognised in survivors of emotional, physical and sexual abuse. In his case, it is of such a severe nature that he loses touch with reality and some of his difficult, aggressive feelings and guilty feelings become expressed as psychotic

phenomena. And that occurs when he's in situations where he feels less supported."

Stigma and discrimination

A few service users talked about being victimised by neighbours, for example being called 'loony' or 'nutter'. One service user said: "a neighbour turned round and said, 'Why are you mad?'", and another service user said:

"The first day I went there [to a new home], there was a letter through my door saying, 'Go back to [the psychiatric hospital] you nutter ... we don't want you here'. But I've had a lot of that kind of stuff."

A consultant said that one service user found just being involved in mental health services was stigmatising and that this was an important reason for why he wanted to withdraw from them. Another service user said that he had initially been unwilling to see a community psychiatric nurse as "that's for nutters", thereby showing his understandable unwillingness to become part of a stigmatised group. Two relatives also mentioned the stigma of mental illness, with one discussing his qualms about using a bus specifically for service users (and staff) to get to one of the psychiatric hospitals:

"I'm going to have get on the bus that all the patients are getting on and what would people think of me? You know, I know it sounds silly ... but there's a stigma to it. You know, by the normal bus not going round anymore they've immediately placed a stigma on the place. And mental illness is still something that isn't accepted."

Context and triggers

The literature on risk assessment and risk management highlights the importance of understanding the triggers that have led to a person becoming a risk to self or others (Grounds, 1995). Many factors can precipitate a psychotic breakdown (Kinderman, 2000) and it was clear from this study that there was a complex interaction between many potentially unhelpful aspects of a person's life that may have increased their chances of experiencing a psychotic breakdown.

"It's sort of like a catch-22 so, when I'm under stress, I tend to hit the bottle quite a bit. I drink a lot so my thought patterns become strange. I become high really when I drink and I start thinking and I start dwelling on the good against the evil again. I start hallucinating...."

Employment is seen as a particularly significant influence on mental health (Warner, 1994; Boardman et al, 2003). Although many service users had been employed in the past, no one was currently in work, and everyone was receiving state benefits and living in poverty. No one had a current long-term relationship or lived with a partner and many people had unsatisfactory or unstable accommodation and had experienced frequent changes in accommodation. Many were homeless at or during admission. Relationship problems, whether with family members, friends, neighbours or co-residents in supported or shared housing were also common, as was social isolation. Some people with dual diagnosis (of mental health and substance misuse) were considered to be exploited, for example 'friends' using the service user's house to take heroin when the service user did not want this to happen. Additional factors mentioned by professionals in relation to risk to self were low self-esteem and having a compulsion to harm oneself to prevent loved ones being harmed.

Other than general stress, not being on medication (or stopping taking it), being unsupported by mental health services and alcohol or substance misuse were seen, by professionals, as having the strongest link with the development of psychosis and problematic behaviour. Service users did not necessarily agree with professionals on these issues. One person thought his poor relationship with a friend was the cause of problems leading to psychiatric service involvement; another said that a vindictive neighbour had caused his problems; another service user denied using alcohol or cannabis while the worker was convinced that he used both and that these were implicated in the deterioration in his mental state; and another person said that his use of amphetamines and some heroin did not affect him adversely.

Taking medication regularly did not prevent breakdown since, although some service users had refused medication or were taking it intermittently, others were regularly taking medication before admission to hospital. Some people stopped taking medication as a consequence of relapse, thinking themselves better or the medication dangerous. Medication is a contentious issue in relation to mental healthcare and it is discussed in some detail in Chapter 6.

Substance misuse was seen by professionals as contributing to the risks, both to the person and to others, in a number of ways. Professionals discussed alcohol or substance use in relation to 13 service users. They were clear that using solvents or amphetamines increased vulnerability to psychosis, dangerous behaviour and risk to physical health. More specific examples included a service user who had nearly died after suffering a respiratory arrest after taking heroin following a break from it due to hospitalisation (resulting in a reduced tolerance to it). Another service user used dirty needles when injecting heroin, something that he only did when experiencing psychosis. Substance misuse also interacted with suicidal tendencies as several service users were considered to pose little risk of suicide unless misusing substances. Professionals saw the effect of alcohol or cannabis as more individual in that it was not considered to have a harmful effect on mental state or behaviour for everyone.

As we shall see in Chapter 5, professionals attempted to address as many of these problems as they could, given available resources, what issues they chose to focus on or prioritise and, significantly, the extent of agreement between themselves and service users about any difficulties.

Summary

While all risk assessment documentation asserts the importance of identifying triggers, many of the service users' lives were so stressful or contained that any one of many unhelpful factors such as poor social circumstances, adverse early experiences, substance misuse, poverty, isolation, or lack of work could have been the trigger for their mental health deteriorating. In their accounts of triggers, professionals were more likely than service users to also mention factors within their remit, that is, use of street drugs or alcohol, involvement with mental health services and use of psychiatric medication. These were the areas with the potential for disagreement between service user and professional.

3

Risk assessment

In this chapter we focus on:

- professionals' views about the impact of defensive practice on risk assessment;
- the methods that they used to assess risk;
- what they found helpful in risk assessment;
- their views about moves towards more formal risk assessments.

Context

'The emphasis is on prioritising people who pose more of a risk and because of the role of secondary mental health services, I mean, we're seeing iller and iller people all the time and that's been a big shift as well in the last few years.... So you get a caseload of 30/35 that are full of the most unwell people, you know, who of course then will attach loads more risk for themselves."

The workers interviewed tended to have considerable professional experience. Most felt reasonably confident about assessing risk while also saying that total confidence was never possible, particularly when trying to reach the right balance between risk taking and risk avoidance:

"But my fear is that I will make a mistake and misread a situation and not respond in time. I mean, I think there are also risks of overreacting and sort of panicking and saying, 'Oh, it's so terrible! We must bundle you straight off to hospital'. And that can also be quite damaging a situation – quite disruptive anyway."

Many also talked about the shift towards more defensive practice within a climate characterised by the following elements: inaccurate media hype about 'mental illness' and dangerousness; a culture of blame where professionals are held accountable, whatever the rights and wrongs of the situation, should anything go wrong; and society's insistence that all risks should be contained and managed.

"So now I think the climate has got much more jumpy.... I think we feel much less able to take clinical risks. And that's a paradox because if you're looking at care in the community, actually there are risks. You cannot make it entirely safe. And if you're not prepared to take calculated risks you're in trouble."

Another worker said:

"Sometimes I think we try to change somebody's circumstances to deal with our own anxieties, rather than the concerns they have about themselves or the risks they actually present."

Confidence was also lower where a person's mental state might deteriorate rapidly, due to heavy use of alcohol or street drugs.

"I think, for us, the combination of the tendency to psychosis and violence and the drug use, somebody living in a situation where we've got very little actual control over whether he attends appointments, whether he takes his medication, whether he uses street drugs, means there is a feeling of responsibility that can't really be delivered in a way. Reality suggests to me that I can't be responsible for this man and what he chooses to do. But I still feel, nonetheless, that, I mean he's on my caseload, I ought to be able to do something more."

Workers were also keenly aware that they were in the difficult area of trying to predict risks accurately so as to manage them. Although research provides information about which groups of people present an increased risk to themselves or others, prediction at the individual level is very difficult. Some hold out the promise of greater predictive ability (MacArthur Research Network, 2001), while others are more pessimistic (Munro and Rumgay, 2000; Petch, 2001). Many professionals talked about the unpredictability of risk assessment:

> "But I think it is *incredibly* difficult to predict which people, particularly when you're dealing with people who are actively psychotic for whom the delusion system can be extremely powerful and very, very frightening. And for those sort of people it is so hard sometimes to know when a paranoia will become so overwhelming that they will strike out."

Many workers and relatives also talked about the impossibility of accurate prediction at the individual level where the risk was to the self. The relatives of several service users, who had talked about the futility of their lives, said that they lived with the constant fear that the person might kill themselves, particularly where they abused substances. A worker also said of one service user: "Every relapse and every time he gets unwell ... he may well just think, 'Well, what's the point?'".

Methods used in risk assessment

The statutory sector

Virtually all professionals said that they constantly assessed risk and discussed it with others working with the service user. Generally speaking, workers were not using standardised or formal methods to assess risk, although nurses on some wards used a form prompting them to tick yes or no to various types of risk, albeit with little space to include context or triggers. Some

considered this useful, while others found it unsophisticated. On some wards these forms were only used once, while on others they were updated and integrated with other professional judgements. In both the hospitals included in the study, discussion about risk took place informally or during handovers between nursing staff, at ward rounds or during care planning meetings. One nurse commented on the difficulty of discussing risks at ward rounds due to time pressures and would have liked a multi-disciplinary forum to discuss risk, which did happen occasionally in other parts of the hospital trust.

The most common method of assessing risk was for workers to use their own mental checklist that included assessing mental state and mood and being aware of past history and factors that they saw as leading to previous breakdown:

> "I just tend to use sort of my own experience and judgement in these situations rather than pro formas and protocols, and that may or may not be a wise thing to do. Probably not a wise thing to do actually."

Others, however, were more systematic:

> "I mean, we have a fairly structured way of looking at people's needs, their functioning and their risks. Yeah. So it does work quite well. And it's reviewed regularly."

Although there was often overlap between the areas that different professionals assessed (for example, the person's current mental state, whether they had intrusive thoughts, and so on), this usually appeared to have happened by chance rather than in a planned way.

The voluntary sector

Some voluntary sector workers commented favourably on the amount of information that they received from referring agencies, while others were less satisfied and had started to develop their own risk assessments as a result of this:

> "Quite often with informal patients in X Hospital there's little or no risk assessment. It might include an informal mention of

risks but it wouldn't be a formalised form of risk assessments and ways of dealing with it. So we're actually in the process here of setting up our own risk assessment but we haven't sort of formalised that yet."

What is helpful in assessing risk?

We asked professionals what was helpful in assessing risk. They most frequently mentioned experience, a good relationship with service users and knowledge of them, including their strengths and abilities, gained over time:

"You can't beat, actually, the hands-on knowledge of what someone is like over a period of time. They're different from seeing someone new for the first time and new to services. Often, you're still being asked to make very similar decisions but with a far less practical background to make those decisions on, and that's where you can make mistakes ... you can misjudge risks or you can just be very unlucky...."

The value of discussion with colleagues, whether that was having a team discussion about risk or jointly assessing risk with colleagues, was also mentioned. However, the extent to which this happened varied considerably. Expected benefits were less subjectivity in risk assessment, less defensive practice, a sharing of responsibility and more creativity in managing risk.

In terms of support, most workers were satisfied with the support that they received from colleagues and immediate managers. However, the majority felt little confidence in senior managers' support to them, should anything go wrong.

Views about a move to formal risk assessment

Many workers knew that more formal methods of risk assessment were being developed. Indeed, towards the end of the research an integrated Care Programme Approach along with standardised risk assessment and management procedures were being developed for use throughout the hospital trust and social services department. Views about whether formal risk

assessment would lead to better decision making varied from enthusiasm to scepticism, particularly from consultant psychiatrists. Indeed, many workers commented on the complexity of risk assessment and how inexact current methods were:

"It's a very defensive process and with very limited scientific backup that formally assessing risk actually does make a difference clinically ... it is a very imprecise science as it is currently outlined."

Some wanted training in risk assessment and management as a way of increasing their confidence. One nurse mentioned the importance of training in techniques to de-escalate aggression and violence, as well as control and restraint as a means of encouraging workers not to reach for extra medication to control a situation.

Most workers were more positive about the potential benefits of moves towards more formal risk assessments, yet they were also concerned about how time-consuming this would be; that it might become bureaucratic form filling to cover professionals' backs without leading to improvements in risk management; and that it might erode the role of judgement and the importance of the relationship with the service user.

"It seems to me that it's gone too far the other way really, where it's become the be-all and end-all ... I mean, I'm not saying you mustn't address these issues, you must, that's good clinical practice. But they mustn't be the drive of the practice."

As another worker said:

"Impression and feel and relationship are important factors in terms of risk, I think, but they're unquantifiable."

Another worry was that formal risk assessment could not fulfil its promise of accurate prediction:

"But these sort of balances between what is risky and what isn't are often perceptions that, from a professional's perspective, can be tarred by lots of different things: litigation; from whether or not you're going to damage the relationship with the person if you overreact, or not react at all. And all those things sort of interact here so the protocols are well and good, it's helpful, but they're only aide memoirs in the end. And they are actually judgements that you make, which are quite complex, I think. And there isn't some sort of standard 'risk assessment objective' structure that will tell you that this person is at risk and you've got to do this, or this person isn't at risk."

One worker talked about how ticking 'yes' items on a risk assessment form, such as 'threats of violence', was unhelpful without other contextual information and that it did not allow the service user's strengths and abilities to be highlighted. Some workers also mentioned concerns about the effects on service users. For example, not allowing for the possibility of change due to the focus on risk factors:

"Although I think formal risk assessments are useful, I still don't think that it's always the case that past behaviour is an indicator of present behaviour and that people shouldn't have the right or the ability to change or evolve – grow, really."

Another issue was that risk assessments could be stigmatising, with the service user seen primarily in terms of their reputation based on behaviour from the distant past that had not been repeated since:

"I've known things that have happened 20 years ago still being repeated about somebody 20 years later. You know, 'This is so-and-so who smashed up such-and-such, or beat up this person or that person'. You know, they've never done it since. You know, they haven't done it in 20 years but it's still something that's being kind of dragged up."

Some also said that risk assessment was being used as a way of excluding people, usually men, from services:

"If they're going to do formal assessments of risks ... and then to use that knowledge to actually manage the risk, not just to say, 'This person is too risky. There's too big a risk. We can't offer them a service'. Which is what my experience has been of other people doing risk assessments – formal risk

assessments.... So, in some ways, I'm glad that we're a bit slow on doing formal risk assessments because we don't say, 'This person's too dangerous for us to work with'. We say, 'How can we work with this person, knowing that there might be some risk?'."

Summary

There was much variation between workers over whether they used systematic or personal methods to assess risk. While some were critical about the ability of risk assessment and management tools to deliver on accuracy, others were more positive. By tools we mean prompts to encourage professionals to comprehensively consider relevant risk factors. No one was using a validated risk assessment instrument[2], which is probably not unusual outside forensic mental health settings. Many workers expressed concern about the impact of adopting more systematic assessment tools on service users, themselves and service quality.

---

[2] That is, validated in the sense that information exists about its success in accurately identifying high and low risk individuals. See Munro (2004) for an excellent account of issues to consider when evaluating the usefulness of risk assessment tools.

4

Discussing risk and reaching agreement

In this chapter we discuss:

- people who were not told that they were considered to pose a potential risk to other people;
- the language used by professionals to discuss risk with service users;
- levels of agreement between professionals and service users about risk;
- service users' and relatives' or friends' knowledge of risk assessment;
- difficulties in establishing the full extent of risk;
- differences in accounts.

Where risk to other people was not discussed with service users

It became clear that some service users could not be asked if they wanted to take part in the research because they were unaware that staff considered them to pose a risk to other people. As one consultant psychiatrist said:

"We may not be as open about our risk assessments as we need to be in order to refer them to the [research] project."

This revealed that some service users were not being involved in trying to reduce risks. Apart from the implications for civil liberties of being placed, without their knowledge, in a stigmatising category and responded to on the basis of perceived risks to others, it meant that a group of people with whom staff have not been frank have been excluded from the study.

Each professional was asked if they worked with any service user who had not been told of professional concerns about risk to other people.

Some said they were always honest while others said that this was something to which they aspired. Many said how difficult it was to discuss risk to others with a service user. Indeed, discussing suicidal intentions was previously seen as encouragement to a person to act on them. Now it is seen as vital to talk to the person about their intentions, including whether they have made a suicide plan (Isacsson and Rich, 2001). Yet a similar body of knowledge about how to discuss risk to others does not exist, nor is there any guidance about how to do this within mental health policy.

Reasons given by professionals in favour of frankness were that it would:

- increase understanding of any triggers;
- help the service user understand the reasons for professional involvement;
- assist in developing a collaborative relationship to minimise risk (albeit that if collaboration was not possible there was always the option of using the 1983 Mental Health Act).

"I think it's more of a risk if it's other people talking about them behind their back. I think the more that things can be out in the open, the less of a risk it is."

Reasons given against frankness were:

- where the service user had no 'insight';
- that the service user would think that the worker was only concerned about risk rather than support or care;
- that the service user would disengage from services;

"And there are people with whom you have tenuous relationships and you don't want to alienate them, so you lose contact with them and you lose the therapeutic relationship, and actually mentioning the fact that they're a risk might cause that."

- discussion would increase feelings of stigma or be harmful to the service user:

"Trying to find a framework in which the client can acknowledge that they represent a risk, without feeling threatened by that acknowledgement, I find quite tricky. For someone to think of themselves as a potential risk.... And the popular media conception, which our clients are just as aware of as anybody else, is that mad people are bad people, are dangerous people."

- fears for the worker's own safety when the service user was psychotic, aggressive or paranoid.

Indeed, the large size of seven service users (all men) was commented on by workers as an aspect of their perceived threat, and seemed to have led to some workers being wary of discussing risk with them:

"He frightens people, you see."

"He's six-foot-three with a menacing appearance."

"He's massive ... he's about six-foot-two and broad shouldered."

One worker had overcome his fears by attending training on risk assessment and management. This had encouraged him to discuss risk with a man described as "quite explosive" who had physically damaged his office:

"I think he was a bit shocked at what I'd said on the risk assessment form. But I went through it with him and he did agree that was how other people might see him, as it were ... and I think, if I can do it with him, I should be able to do it with anybody."

He added:

"And I think that it's interesting that, since we did that risk assessment, he's been much better with us.... You know, I sometimes think it may have improved his relationship with us."

This example is important as it shows that this professional's fears about frank discussion of risk were not realised. In fact, openness resulted in less aggression and a better working relationship. Sometimes people with mental health problems are not tackled about their behaviour because of fears about personal safety or concerns that they may need to be protected from aspects of themselves or be incapable of change.

The language used to discuss risk

The first step in developing a risk management plan with service users is discussion of risk. Most professionals said that they did this:

"... and if we can't, then we need to increase our skill and knowledge base about how it is we talk about those things with people."

Another stressed her responsibility:

"I think they need to know so that, you know, if they're becoming unwell, they have a choice then. I think, up to a certain point, these people have a responsibility to say, 'I'm a bit unwell'. But, then, I think that we go past that point. So it gives them a choice I think."

There was also a fear of the potential harm to the person's sense of self as well as a reluctance to stigmatise them by labelling them as dangerous:

"I mean, my experience of anybody, not with X but with other people who have similar problems, is that one of the most disabling things about those acute phases is that people can think, behave and act in ways that, under normal circumstances (whatever 'normal' is) they wouldn't dream of doing so."

Professionals found it difficult to discuss behaviour with people who downplayed or denied that any grounds for concern existed or who were mortified by their behaviour and found it difficult to acknowledge an aspect of themselves that they found so alien and unwelcome. Some staff mentioned the difficulty of discussion with people who had no recollection of what they have done and where telling them would make them feel ashamed. Many professionals were at pains to point out to us the positive qualities of service users. It was clear that they valued the person and could see beyond their behaviour when unwell. For example:

"He's actually quite a caring person."

"… quite a gentle person really."

"It's clear, seeing him with other patients, how he tries to help other people."

The fact that ordinary, peaceful and caring people can change their character during a mental health crisis, either because they feel threatened or voices tell them to behave in particular ways, is of course well known within mental health circles. Yet such knowledge is seldom included in the literature about risk and dangerousness. The issue of this discrepancy between behaviour in crisis compared with their 'true' character might be a source of discussion about understanding of the effects of psychosis on an otherwise peaceful person. This might help a service user to feel more understood rather than controlled.

> Good practice suggestion: Workers could try to talk with *all* service users identified as a risk to others about the effects of psychosis on their identity and behaviour, while also acknowledging their strengths and abilities.

It was clear in the tentativeness of the language used by some workers, for example, "I *try* to discuss risk with him", that full and frank discussion was an area of difficulty. Sometimes this was due to the service user's unwillingness to discuss risk, although it could also be due to the quality of relationship between a specific worker and service user. One ward manager, who had known a service user over a long period, discussed with him how he frightened other people, whereas other staff were wary of doing so:

"So he would actually talk to me a little bit more than most people. And I think the problem with X is that a lot of people were quite scared of him. You know, if you actually spoke to him about things, he was actually OK."

One worker commented that discussion about risk could sometimes be a "little bit coy", and another said:

"I mean, I don't like to use terms like 'risk' in that sense, but I mean I think he does accept that there are concerns about his behaviour."

While another said:

"Risk to others particularly, it's not something that's necessarily as openly addressed as it might be. We tend to use things like 'early warning signs' and 'relapse indicators'."

Some workers directly told service users how their behaviour affected others, for example, "Do you know you're frightening people?", and the effect could be profound:

"I don't think he does realise how menacing he can be…. But I still think, genuinely, he still is quite horrified by the fact that people may find him to be scary."

There was awareness of the impact of such an unwanted message. A voluntary sector manager said:

"And sometimes I say things which are hard for people to hear."

Some service users may not have been clear that they were perceived by professionals to be a risk to others. This is difficult territory. It could be argued that it is not helpful for professionals to use the language of risk with service users or tell them that they consider them to pose a potential risk to themselves or others. Indeed, some professionals were keenly aware of how stigmatising such judgements and language could be. Anecdotal evidence was also provided by one professional (not involved in the study) who had given a service user a copy of a risk assessment that concluded that he was at high risk of suicide. The professional said that a close family member was convinced that seeing this assessment had been a significant factor in the person's subsequent suicide.

Yet how can this potential risk be balanced with the fact that it can be argued that it is a civil rights issue that service users should know that this is how they are being defined, and therefore being responded to, by professionals?

Good practice suggestion: There is a pressing need for discussion between mental health service user groups and professionals on the topic of how best to discuss risks and how to inform service users when professionals consider them to pose a potential risk to others. This should include the real and perceived benefits and disadvantages of being open with service users about risk.

Level of agreement

Since the 1983 Mental Health Act can be used to ensure compliance with treatment, agreement is not necessary for professional involvement. However, it is generally felt that relationships between service user and professional are more likely to be effective where there is agreement about risk.

> "Obviously, if they can acknowledge that there is a problem then we're in a much better position to ensure that they put something in place which works."

The research suggested that professionals were most confident when service users agreed with their professional opinion. Much effort was directed at getting the service user to agree about risks, although the term 'risk' was not necessarily used. Some professionals tried to understand how service users viewed risks and were willing to move some direction away from what they thought was ideal in order to accommodate the service user. However, the more dangerous the behaviour was to other people, the less room for manoeuvre professionals had to accommodate the service user's perspective where this conflicted with their professional opinion.

Agreement between professional and service user ranged from complete agreement to none at all. Seven service users were open to discussing risk, were clear with professionals that their behaviour

had been a risk to others and accepted the care plan put into place to manage risk.

One man said that, when hearing voices, he would sometimes obtain a sharp weapon and think about killing a mental health worker or fellow resident whom he believed would harm him. He always made this situation clear to mental health workers and handed over his weapons on request. All the mental health workers' accounts of his behaviour agreed completely with his own.

> "And I said, 'Look, I'm going to kill someone in this house tonight or something, or in the next few nights, if you don't get me out of here'."

While not denying the seriousness of the potential threats, staff working with this man also saw this as a cry for help, as the service user said:

> "I think if you asked Dr X, he [would] probably say that me pulling a knife was me saying 'help'."

Several service users told us openly that they had harmed or threatened others and how much distress their behaviour caused them:

> "You know when I start getting towards the point when I, myself, am getting violent.... I don't know what I would do with myself if I had hit X. You know, even if the injuries hadn't been severe, I still don't know what I what I would have done with myself."

Both the women in the research study spoke openly about the major risk that they posed to others and one said:

> "And the thing that worries me is that when I'm in that state of mind it is logical to take the children with me. I could not leave them with the burden of a mother who killed herself ... and when my thinking gets like that I need to be away from them because in that state of mind they are just extensions of me."

However, some workers thought that agreement might be difficult to maintain if the service user became 'unwell'.

With five service users there was little or no agreement with professionals. Attempts to discuss risk with one service user were described as:

"Very difficult. Very difficult. He'll deny many of the incidents that I've told you about. He'll say that the police are wrong, that they were harassing him. That he didn't do these things. That he's not a risk to other people.... So it's very, very difficult, yeah, to find any middle ground there really."

Attempting to find the 'middle ground' was exploring with the service user how their behaviour might be misunderstood by others. Even this level of discussion was not possible with two service users who, according to staff, would either become irate or walk out. With one service user there were also fears about personal safety, since he had committed some 'fairly serious assaults' without warning. One of the service users who had, according to staff, made serious threats when unwell said, in response to a question about whether he felt that he could be a risk to other people:

"I've never harmed anybody and I've never done anything. In the years I've been coming to hospital all I do is help other people."

The other service users fell somewhere between the two extremes of agreement, for example, where risk was discussed but its seriousness not fully agreed or where the person was unable (due to perceived cognitive deficits) or unwilling to fully discuss their behaviour or their mental state. Indeed, some service users in this group told us that they had thoughts that that they would not tell professionals.

Overall, there was only one person who completely denied to us that they had ever behaved in any ways which had ever frightened or threatened other people. Everyone else described to us behaviour that was frightening, even if, as in the following example, they did not agree with workers' opinions about being a risk to others:

"I've never harmed anybody and I've never done anything in the last nine years since I've been coming to hospital."

But this service user also said:

"I threatened the doctor seven years ago. It was because he said I had to have injections."

Knowing the service user over time and valuing their qualities was seen by professionals as important in creating optimum conditions in which to discuss risk. They also felt that service users needed to feel that they, as professionals, had their interests at heart rather than being only concerned with risk:

"And, you know, if I hadn't known X so well I probably would have been careful. But because I knew him quite well I could be quite specific and quite direct."

Timing was seen as particularly important with concerns that raising the subject when the person was experiencing psychosis was counter-productive and possibly dangerous:

"... if, after a certain point in his illness, I reflect it back to him the way he was behaving, you know, and I voice my concerns, I don't know what response I'd get."

There was little evidence of formal discussions about risk or of risk assessments being completed involving the service user, although some workers talked about its importance. One social worker said that this was regrettably "usually done behind closed doors". Another worker said:

"You know, I think it's very disempowering for professionals to simply carry out a risk assessment if you're not involving the service user in it.... I don't know how much they are involved in it. I mean, I think *I try* to involve my service users if I'm concerned about some risk."

A small number of professionals said that they thought that service users were less involved in discussing risk where the risk was to others rather than to themselves.

Good practice example: In two voluntary organisations, service users were fully involved in discussions about risk. Additionally, in one of the organisations, service users completed the referral form with a worker. The form asked them for information about risks to themselves or to other people.

In contrast with the variety of levels of agreement between service users and professionals about risk, levels of agreement both between professionals and between relatives and professionals were high.

Service users' and relatives' or friends' knowledge of risk assessment

"They've got an opinion on you. They've got an opinion on your risk. They write down all about your illness and you're being assessed. But it's all done by writing. Do you know what I mean? There's no verbal communication really."

Overall, service users were not given copies of any risk assessments that had been carried out and they were not always told that one had been done, although many workers wanted to work towards this. One service user said that he had seen all his risk assessments. However, there is some doubt about this as, according to him, all reports described him as not a risk. Three service users assumed that a risk assessment had been done, with one saying:

"I don't know if anyone was trying to assess risk with me. Ah, let me think. Well Dr X would obviously be trying to keep some angle on that. But [Dr X] didn't really ask me too many open questions."

The other service users said that they didn't know whether any risk assessments had been done.

The only time that service users had seen copies of any reports that discussed risk were when they had gone to a Mental Health Review Tribunal to try and get their sections removed. All three of the service users to which this applies were unhappy about some aspects of the report – one person in particular at what he

considered to be inaccuracy about his ability to live independently. Another service user said that no one had discussed with him the fact that his report described him as a risk to himself and others.

Of the friends and relatives, one assumed that risk assessments had been conducted, while the others said that they did not know. One relative talked about their disappointment about the lack of a risk assessment as the service user, when unwell, could be extremely threatening to them. Another relative said:

"They didn't have a particular meeting about the risks, but they did say, if he came home, that would be a risk."

He added:

"If they did [do a risk assessment], then they should talk to me."

Good practice example: A community-based consultant psychiatrist and community psychiatric nurse had started to jointly assess risk for all service users. They had decided to do this without involving the service users but were planning to discuss their joint assessments with them at care plan meetings:

"I guess, in a way, we'll have our agenda and then, when that's sorted out, look with the client about what the risks are. But I think, with the risk assessments, it seems good that we can actually sit back and have a look at the situation ourselves, as professionals, and see what areas we need to be managing, really, but then feed that back at the care programme."

Good practice example: One professional had just started using their trust's newly developed risk assessment and management forms. The service user had been given a risk assessment summary sheet with the main risk factors. The care plan meeting had openly discussed the risks that he posed to others, and he had been given a verbal account of a risk assessment, which he said he 'didn't mind'.

Difficulties in establishing the full extent of risk: gaps in knowledge and information sharing

There were worrying gaps in knowledge about the accounts of service user behaviour among professionals interviewed and indeed, some workers mentioned it as a problem. Examples were given of people admitted or discharged with little information provided to relevant workers about risk or how to manage it. Staff working with the same service user did not always have access to previous risk assessments and a few were unsure whether any risk assessment had been carried out. Not having accessible information about risk was of concern to many workers:

"The most worrying patients are the ones with four volumes of notes and it's known that in the past they did something worrying. But trying to find out and what were the circumstances around it.... Because, as I say, it isn't so important what they did, it's what the circumstances around it were, and that's what's difficult to find out. And you can't make future plans if you don't know that detail. And to do a proper risk assessment takes a lot of time: of just sitting down with four volumes of notes and just raking through it."

We asked professionals about where on the service user's file information about risk could be found. This was not usually in a specific section but spread throughout a file. Relevant information could be in the care plan, on care management review forms, in discharge summaries or letters to GPs. Indeed, when staff referred to case notes during the interview, they sometimes had to rifle through pages of information to find accounts of risk factors. One person described the process as "hunting through the file". Many commented on how time-consuming it was to find relevant information. One worker had done a risk assessment that he said should be at the front of the file but which had become "buried in all the correspondence". Information could be contained in several volumes of files, with the most current one not always having a historical summary:

"You know, it's very annoying when you find somebody's notes, they've got a new volume opened and there's virtually nothing in it, yet you know there's three or four previous volumes with stacks of information on them which, of course, have been archived in Medical Records. But an electronic system will sort [that out]."

In the most worrying case, a doctor, who had met a certain service user once, was unable to find any record of risk factors within the case notes. He found a discharge summary that said "risk factors had already been well documented". That may have been the case, but they were not in the current file.

This echoes findings elsewhere in research evaluating the use of supervision registers in England:

For a surprising number of supervision registers cases there was little evidence in case notes or from staff about actual incident of harm, despite the importance of such incidents for risk assessment. (Thornicroft, 2000)

We also found that information was commonly spread across different files, for example community psychiatric nurse files, social work records, day hospital files and in-patient records.

"And if we write on those set[s] of notes and then he gets admitted, they disappear to X hospital. And he might only be in for a few days but the notes get lost. So we're seeing him without seeing, maybe, what has been written when he's been in hospital."

One social worker commented that if the service user said something worrying to her, she could tell colleagues but they would not necessarily note this in their records. The files that her team used did not have any markers to alert colleagues to potential risks, particularly important if she was away from the office.

Good practice example: Some mental health services were moving towards one file for service users with a specific section for risk assessments. A few workers had written a summary of past risk and a community-based team was developing a summary of risk information for each service user with information from both community psychiatric nurse and medical files together:

> "Starting with the patients we believe are at highest risk, we're trying to work through the whole caseload, or as much of it as we need to, to actually formalise and document the risk assessment."

Good practice suggestion: It might be useful to reserve and mark clearly a specific place within case notes for an account of risk behaviour. This could include the chronology of incidents[3], the context within which they took place, as well as information on issues such as weapons used, verbal threats made, and so on. Such information should be transferred when a new volume of notes is started. Additionally, it might be useful to discuss this information with the service user, who should also receive a copy of it, in order to ascertain their views about the information, as well as provide an account – from their point of view – of the pressures that they were experiencing at the time. This would help to establish the accuracy of any summary about past risk.

Differences in accounts

Risk to others

There are several reasons why having accurate information is important. Professionals clearly have to balance the rights of patients not to be restricted more than necessary with the rights of others not to be harmed. However, getting a good balance and assessing changes in behaviour over time become problematic without detailed and accurate information. There is also

the right of service users to have accurate information about them on record since, otherwise, life-long harm can be done to people's reputations, particularly as it is commonly asserted that the most accurate predictor of future behaviour is previous episodes of threat and harm.

While there was much consistency in the accounts given by all our informants, we were also given information by service users about risk to others which staff did not mention and vice versa. Interestingly, a worker in one of the two voluntary organisations where risk was more openly discussed said that this had led to some service users volunteering previously unknown information about risk.

We also found examples of conflicting descriptions of behaviour. For example, one worker said that he had "heard" that a service user had hit someone with a hammer, while everyone else, including the service user, described a different weapon and no physical harm. Another service user said that he had "grabbed the doctor by the collar", whereas the ward keyworker said that he had "tried to strangle the consultant". A threatened stabbing (not mentioned by the service user in question) was described by one professional as a risk factor, while another said:

> "He's been accused of going to stab a staff member. I was present on that occasion and it was very half-hearted. It was with one of our table knives and he came in waving it. And there was no way he was going to stick it in him. But that's gone down as an attempted stabbing."

Records for another service user said that he had "attacked" a doctor and a healthcare worker, although other information suggested that they were the same person. His account was of threatening a doctor wanting to inject him and that he had no weapon with him. As with all these examples, the service user was unaware that his record showed that he had attacked someone. The account gave no information about context, which is crucial in terms of assessing risk, or the service user's views about why the situation had arisen:

---

[3] See Stanley and Manthorpe (2001) for a discussion of the importance of chronological accounts of risk.

"In his file it said that he was transferred to X Hospital from Y Hospital because he assaulted a healthcare worker. But that's all it says."

Length of time since assaults or other types of harm is significant in trying to establish whether risk is decreasing or not. Accounts of one service user having assaulted someone "years ago" contradicted another worker saying that this had happened "in the last couple of admissions, *apparently*" (our emphasis).

Sometimes there was agreement about what had happened, but not about its seriousness. For example, one service user thought that his behaviour had been "unwise" rather than a serious risk. Professionals were more concerned but still unsure about the level of seriousness:

"There was an assumption, for want of better information really, that if it had been a serious assault, the police would have been involved."

This service user was one of four whose behaviour was seen as threatening to neighbours. The service users saw themselves as being provoked to defend themselves rather than making unprovoked threats. For some, so many incidents were reported that a picture of serious risk emerged. However, where service users disagreed and accounts were vague, conflicting, second- or even third-hand, it was difficult for professionals to assess the seriousness of behaviour. For example, professionals working with one man thought that he had opened his door, holding a knife, to a neighbour. They agreed that this was due to him feeling threatened, with no *objective* grounds for feeling this way. However:

"On his discharge summary it says that he actually went to the neighbour's front door. Which is actually quite different in terms of him approaching her rather than her approaching him. So, I suppose, the first thing that I thought was that he was hearing these voices and that he'd actually come to his door and that he'd been frightened and that he'd come to the door with a knife. But, now, I'm not so sure really."

Attempts to find out what had really happened were difficult because the service user was "evasive about the whole thing". The differing accounts revolved around whether this service user was being threatening or trying to protect himself (albeit in a threatening way) due to fear. Trying to establish the truth would be highly significant in terms of risk management but seemed impossible.

Additionally, it seemed that although the police had been involved in some incidents involving service users in this study, workers did not receive any written information from them. For example, a worker knew that there had been two incidents leading to the service user being arrested and sectioned but did not know the full details of what had happened, and therefore how serious the risk was.

Good practice suggestion: Incidents that might be relevant in assessing risk to other people need to be quickly and clearly documented.

This might include all of the following:

- Questioning witnesses.
- Requesting a copy or summary of police records where there has been police involvement. Allowance should be made for the possibility that the police may not take the service user's accounts of what has happened as seriously as if they were not seen as 'mentally ill'.
- Two staff, one of them a manager, signing the account to ensure that it is detailed properly.
- Showing the account to the service user so that they understand what has been written and to add their own explanation about what happened to the record.

In making the above suggestion, we do not discount the impact of the assaults and threats on those who received them. Nor do we suggest that either staff or service user accounts are always the 'correct' ones. But the date and nature of such events should be clear if risk assessments are to be improved and accurate.

Risk to self

While much information about risk to self was known, in some cases it was inaccurate or not shared between relevant people. A few workers failed to mention past suicide attempts or self-harm. For example, one service user's friend was the only person to say that he had tried to hang himself. One consultant confidently asserted that a service user never thought about suicide while the service user, relative and keyworker all thought that he was a suicide risk during admission, although the hospital notes gave no information about this:

> "I think with this thing, unfortunately, when people are well it tends to get forgotten, unfortunately."

The relative was also the only person to describe the service user as a suicide risk during the weeks after discharge, a time associated with a high risk of suicide (Harris and Barraclough, 1997). One service user had been frank about his suicidal ideas and was perplexed about the lack of response from services:

> "But I've never been, like, considered a serious risk to my own health, which is a bit strange 'cos I've talked to them about suicide before and they know I'm really pissed off about things in here."

One keyworker thought that a service user no longer heard voices telling him to kill himself whereas the service user said that he experienced them constantly. Two service users disclosed prior sexual abuse to the interviewer, something which no one else mentioned. Indeed, one person's self-destructive behaviour, mentioned by only one of the professionals working with him, fitted the profile of someone who had been sexually abused. (Chapter 5 gives examples of practice with service users where workers knew about sexual abuse.)

Structured discussion of risk, information sharing and accurate record keeping would help avoid these worrying gaps in information.

Good practice suggestion: To be effective, a risk assessment should:

- discuss and record *all* risks with service users (including self-harm, sexual abuse, exploitation, stigma, racism and discrimination), not just risk to others;
- establish the accuracy of information;
- describe the context of risk;

- include the service user's account and explanation;
- assess the seriousness of any risk, as well as how long ago it happened.

For risk assessment and management to work well, there needs to be accurate information about the level and likelihood of risk to others. Information about risks tends to be based on professional accounts, yet this research shows these accounts and information held in case records can be vague, missing or contradictory.

In a few cases, community staff were unaware that some service users had behaved in ways that caused risk to others when in hospital. One worker said:

> "As far as I'm aware, there is no risk to other people. I don't know anything on his records which would indicate that."

Although this service user was seen as more of a risk to himself, ward staff and workers who knew him before admission to hospital also saw him as a threat to others. Another worker interviewed a service user alone in the community only to discover later that hospital staff would not see him alone:

> "I received a referral for X from Dr Y and there was no mention of any risk in this letter."

One ward keyworker had also experienced difficulty in getting information about a service user's stay in another hospital, which he saw as unusual.

Good practice suggestion: Information-sharing protocols could help to ensure that information about risk is passed to relevant staff and includes information about risk behaviour on hospital wards and whether or not a person should be seen alone.

Summary

While we found examples of good practice in discussing risk, this chapter shows that some people were not aware that they were considered by professionals to pose a potential risk to other people. The interviews with professionals explored the reasons why they felt honesty was not always achievable. Whether the word 'risk' was actually used emerged as another area of variation between professionals. This is an issue that demands further discussion between professionals and mental health service user groups. Our own view is that service users should always know when professionals consider that they may pose a potential risk to other people. Timing is, however, important: service users should not be told when experiencing a psychotic period where discussion about risk would exacerbate their distress.

This chapter shows differing levels of agreement between service users and professionals about risk, ranging from unanimous agreement to little or none, something that has clear implications for how acceptable service users will find risk management plans and the involvement of mental health professionals in their lives. Agreement between professionals and relatives or friends was much closer. Service users and relatives/friends tended not to know that risk assessments had been completed, although there were some examples of user involvement in assessing risk to others and to self.

While some risks were shared and agreed with everyone concerned, other risk information was either unknown or inaccurate. This led to distortion about levels of risk, with implications for service users, professionals and others. Underestimation of risk could lead to service users being under-supported, as well as to professionals and others being at risk. Overestimation of risk could lead to the service user developing an unwarranted reputation for being dangerous and being responded to on that basis by agencies with whom they come into contact.

Not only is doing a risk assessment without accurate information like building a house without proper foundations, but it also reduces the likelihood of developing effective risk management plans.

5

Care planning and risk assessment and management

In this chapter, we discuss:

- how professionals managed risk;
- care planning and service users' views about the process, including their involvement and influence;
- the support offered to service users[4];
- service users' views about care plans and support;
- delays in support;
- relatives' and friends' views of support;
- support not offered;
- relationships, communication, continuity of care and ethical dilemmas.

When leaving hospital, care plans for support in the community were made under the Care Programme Approach (CPA). All but one service user had formal CPA meetings, with many service users under section 117 of the 1983 Mental Health Act. All the care plans included the way in which risks were going to be managed in the community. The technical aspects of planning support or setting up a care plan give rise to jargon, which may conceal that decisions about the person's lifestyle and their quality of life are being made.

How professionals managed risk

Good practice in risk management suggests that it should be an integral part of care and be based upon planning for individuals (Morgan, 1999). It is an accurate assessment of:

- mental state
- past behaviour
- social functioning
- social circumstances.

Although it was clear that professionals took these factors into account, overall this was not done formally. It was rare for there to be a written risk management or relapse plan and a few professionals said that risk assessment was emphasised at the expense of risk management. Perhaps because workers had no method to systematically manage risk it was difficult to clearly identify risk management strategies as opposed to general care planning.

Where care plan forms were used, they varied as to how much information they contained about risk and its management and whether service users were given written information about risk. One psychiatrist, who discussed risk with *most* service users, expressed concern about service users being given information:

"I think the problem comes with things like the care programming, you know, because you have to define what the risk is.... You have to say whether you think they're a risk, you know, to themselves, to others or, you know, self-neglect. And you have to put that down quite candidly, you know, quite openly and they get a copy of that. And you have to be quite clear about why you've done it. And I know some people don't like it. And, you know, I think it makes clients think that that's all you're interested in doing."

He also feared what the service user might say or do:

---

[4] Chapter 6 focuses in some detail on two major forms of 'support': medication and housing.

"'Oh, doctor, you've written this on this form and you say I'm a risk to others and I'm not and I'm coming down to sort you out'."

During the study, the mental health trust developed risk assessment and management forms to integrate with care plans. The new care plans had information about risk factors and signs of relapse and the review of the care plan included a section for the service user's views about the plan. One professional began using these forms during the study and considered risk formally every time there was a CPA. He discussed risk with the service user but did not give him a copy because:

"I think that it would not be very constructive for X to see these sort of checklist-type documents about him. I think these are things which are helpful for professionals but not constructive for him."

While he did not elaborate on the reasons for this comment, it may be that he was concerned about the impact on service users of being given information suggesting that they are a risk to themselves or other people. He did say, however, that he would be interested in finding out whether service users would find it helpful to have copies of risk assessments.

In general, professionals were reasonably confident that risk would be managed and therefore minimised if they:

- could provide the level of support they thought necessary;
- could ensure that the service user took medication;
- had a good relationship and regular contact with the service user;
- had effective communication with other professionals.

Although there were also individually tailored aims, the care plan for every service user included monitoring mental health and encouraging compliance with medication. Care coordinators and psychiatrists were more confident about managing risk when the service user was also seen regularly by other workers, such as daycare, drop-in or housing support workers. For example, one psychiatrist was no longer so concerned about a service user, who had been admitted in extreme circumstances, because of his willingness to accept services and take medication. Other situations were more worrying:

"I feel that we're kind of doing the best we can. But I think there are situations where the assessment is difficult; we might not have all the information; the patient may not be as open with us as we need; perhaps there aren't enough resources going into the situation, for whatever reason, and inevitably, then, the confidence is much lower."

Agreement about risk management between service users and professionals was a significant issue and where lacking, workers were understandably less confident about managing risk. Talking generally, one worker commented on forensic risk assessments that documented risk but where:

"Nobody's really got any real idea about how to manage it in the context of somebody who can't be forced to receive services."

Involvement and influence at care plan meetings

A distinction needs to be made between service user involvement and influence at care plan meetings. For example, when professionals talked about someone being 'involved', some meant this to be that the service user had expressed their views (which may or may not have been taken into account), while others meant that they had actually influenced the outcome. The following account illustrates professional confusion:

"But then, when a decision has been made, right, as a case coordinator, I have to say, 'Look X, we had a meeting yesterday, you were supposed to be here but you weren't'.... And I'll say, 'OK. This is what was decided. Right?'. I say. 'I want you to take your medication regularly, and come and see me once a week'. Yes. So they are involved. They are involved."

As one service user said:

"They was telling me what was going to happen."

A small number of service users were considered involved and were seen as articulate about what they wanted from the care plan:

"He's intelligent and articulate and contributes well to the care plan."

"I think in his last care plan he was quite involved really about telling us when he was feeling unsafe and about how he felt was the best way to communicate his feelings."

One service user said:

"I felt involved because I seem to get on with the psychiatrists and the doctors. They seem to be on my sort of wavelength really. No, no, I feel quite easy with them. I tell them that I do want be involved.... I want to know exactly what the plans are for myself."

Few professionals discussed how to involve people who were not forthcoming about the support that they wanted, although one social worker described the issue:

"But it's very sad because he's always so pleased and grateful for everything and you always have to say to him, 'Look this had to be your decision.... but I think something has happened along the way where he feels very worthless."

Checking with the service user about whether they feel that they are involved and/or have any influence might reveal differences between the professional and the service user, for example, between the doctor who thought that the service user was happy with the care plan ("We come to sort of a mutually agreeable thing.") and the service user's view that being offered daycare and the chance to talk to a professional whom he had little faith in was not much of a care plan.

Good practice example: A voluntary sector housing provider encouraged tenants to draw up their own care plans and provided assistance to do so.

Service users' ability to be involved or influential in care plan meetings was also seen by professionals as depending on their mental state:

"When he's reasonably well adjusted he can talk about, you know, activity or, you know, talk about his behaviour. It depends really on whether he's well mentally or whether he's in a sort of crazy, paranoid state, really."

Only one service user had a legal advocate at a care plan meeting to press for housing. No one else had an advocate at meetings and no worker, except one, mentioned that involving an advocate might have encouraged some service users to express their views. This worker said that an advocate might have been helpful for a service user who was rejecting his care plan:

"And I think he might feel better about somebody totally empathising with him and putting forward his point of view at a care programme meeting."

Some professionals were unaware that service users whom they were working with were critical of their care plans.

Good practice suggestions:

- Encourage service users to draw up advance directives so that their opinion about what works best for them, including their views about medication, can be taken into account should they experience a period of mental distress in the future.
- Give service users information about independent advocacy services.
- Be flexible about the number of people attending care plan meetings in order to enable service users to be involved.
- Offer the service user the support and preparation time they need to attend care plan meetings. If the service user does not attend, the CPA care coordinator should ensure that the user's views are represented and feedback is given to them.

For some service users in the study the stress involved in meeting large numbers of professionals at care plan meetings, some of whom they did not know, was a barrier to their involvement. One service user asked for extra medication before his meeting and another service user decided not to attend. His worker, who attended on his behalf, said:

"I mean, I'd feel very nervous and that people were judging me if I was in a room full of, you know, other professionals sort of making judgements on my life.... So it was sort of a bit of advocacy for X, to raise the points for him."

Support offered to service users

Research shows (Kinderman, 2000) that attention to a person's psychosocial needs, whether for adequate housing, valued work or for talking therapy can powerfully affect mental health. As one worker stated:

"I mean, because I construct risk [management] within the context of the social system that people live in. The way that we work is that we try to provide as supportive a social structure as is possible outside of here so that, when the people leave here, we look for appropriate settings."

Although not all service users agreed to the following, at discharge they were offered:

- regular appointments with a psychiatrist;
- attending a group, daycare or a drop-in facility;
- medication (for some service users).

With the exception of two people, everyone was also in contact with a mental health professional such as a community psychiatric nurse or social worker.

Other support provided included:

- social activities for people with a dual diagnosis;
- intensive rehabilitation services;
- psychological help or psychotherapy;
- help with finding accommodation;
- assistance in maintaining a tenancy;
- help with finding employment, daytime or leisure activities such as drama and art courses.

An intensive support team to reduce the risk of readmission was used for some service users. Referral to a psychologist or to a psychotherapy group for issues such as managing voices encouraging harm to others, sexual abuse, vulnerability to sexual exploitation or low self-esteem was also used. One service user had been assisted by the mental health services to the point of prosecution of the perpetrator of abuse, although the prosecution had then been dropped.

One service user completed a questionnaire about voices with his community psychiatric nurse and he said: "It gives me insight into myself". The psychiatrist of another service user was also helping him manage his auditory hallucinations.

One man was involved in a Patient's Council and two others had been encouraged to refer themselves to self-help groups, although neither had felt able to do this.

Although professionals are clearly in a more powerful position than service users, many said that they negotiated with service users to try and reach a mutually acceptable care plan. Several discussed the ineffectiveness of trying to impose a care plan without agreement. However, the legal enforcement of treatment has a powerful effect on the leeway service users have to negotiate. One worker said that if the service user was unhappy about the proposals for support, "we'll explore why and look at alternatives *if it is felt appropriate*" (our emphasis).

Service users' views about care plans and support

Service users did not discuss support in terms of risk management and only a few were explicitly told that it was being provided in order to deal with the risks that they were seen as presenting. They were not always aware that risk assessment and management was an integral aspect of a worker's role.

Good practice suggestion: Inform all service users that assessing and managing risk is an integral part of the role of mental health workers.

Half the service users felt that they were getting a reasonable level of support (sometimes for the first time, despite previous hospital admissions). One service user who saw professional help at Phase 1 as "interference" was happy with the support provided after discharge. He described it as being to make sure that he was safe, take his medication and look after himself. He also said:

"Yeah, it's definitely better than not having them, really, because you can sort of ring them up and say, 'Listen. I don't feel so good', and they'll probably say, 'Yeah, well, I'll pop round then' or something like that. Just to check up on you."

Another service user had moved into supported accommodation and was receiving support from a community psychiatric nurse, housing support worker, doctor and social worker:

"They'll probably check up on me, make sure I'm taking my medication, and sticking with my course, and keeping on an even keel towards a full recovery (I suppose is the way they put it)."

Another service user said:

"I think with the resources they've got available, they do a good job."

Only a handful of service users were fully involved in relapse plans but one of these service users said that he had found it really helpful. His comments show that he felt supported by his doctor since, at the first interview, he had said:

"Everything that they think about me and everything about my clinical illness is all written in those notes. They've got an opinion on you. They've got an opinion on your risk. They write down all about your illness and you're being assessed. But it's all done by writing. There's no verbal communication, really."

Whereas at the second interview he commented:

"Yeah, he seemed quite concerned. He wanted to help. He wanted to look back in my past history and try and find out the best ways of dealing with it, really."

> Good practice example: This service user and his doctor spent some months going through his file to assess risk and develop a management plan. The service user and others, including his family, had a letter detailing what to do if he became unwell. It also provided contact names. This made him more confident about getting a quicker response than previously, should he become psychotic.

Unfortunately the doctor subsequently moved, leaving the service user unsure if the next one would accept the plan. He was concerned about this since he had previously experienced many changes of doctor. Although he had a relapse plan, he did not feel that well supported:

"It's like another one of these great ideas from the NHS, isn't it? You've got, like, a care plan, what a great idea. But does it actually work because it breaks down all the time? There's so much emphasis put on something that, in theory, is going to work. But, in reality, again it breaks down and the people who are involved in your care plan are not there anymore. So who takes over the reins?"

Other service users were not necessarily asking for more support from mental health services but wanted "a better environment" or to be less lonely and the following comment suggests some disillusionment with the care plan:

"I didn't know what they was on about with a care plan. What care plan? Is it a care plan to go to X every so often? Go to X, have a drug test and a chat."

Other service users agreed to some but not all of the care plan, for example accepting support with accommodation but not wanting to take medication or refusing to give up street drugs. Other service users had no choice as they were still under section and a few wanted more support than they were offered or found that the support that they had valued had been withdrawn.

There was little sense that service users were aware of, or involved in, choice about the full range of potential services. It seemed that professionals offered the services that they thought would be helpful rather than an informed choice being made by service users.

Good practice suggestion: Service users should be given accessible information (for example, in leaflet form) about:

- the range of services available within mental health services;
- self-help strategies and psychological approaches to mental distress;
- mental health service policy, including responses to crises and relapse plans.

However, knowing about services does not necessarily mean that service users will receive them. A few talked about having no influence over the withdrawal of services that they still wanted. One service user, promised a high level of support at discharge, was refused extra support, which he found infuriating:

"Ultimately I feel penalised because I can hold it together for a very very long time and it's just like they'll let me, they'll let me hold it together until it falls apart."

He was the only service user who did not get the extra help that he asked for. His needs came within the remit of different social work teams with separate eligibility criteria. He was also not considered to have 'a serious mental illness' and so was refused additional psychiatric services.

"I'm probably not psychotic enough for a CPN, obviously. I mean, I could go there. I mean, probably, eventually I will if the pressure keeps up with no support. You know, I'll end up where I was last year, [that is, hospital] as much as I don't want to and as much as I'm putting it off."

This is a worrying example of someone needing and wanting more support to reduce the chance of a crisis developing that could put himself and others at risk.

"I realise everybody's hands are tied by limited funding ... but it seems a false economy to me because, if this goes the whole nine yards, then I'm going to be back to Middletown Hospital and they're going to be paying for me staying in there.... And, to me, it just seems a bit

odd. And that was one of the things, you know, I was quite interested in about the project."

The service user's worker said that the National Health Service Framework's focus on people with a serious mental illness, "by which they mean psychotics wielding a knife", had led to mental health services being unwilling to provide the additional support needed.

Delays in support

The following comment from a service user's friend illustrates the critical importance of an effective response:

"There's people out there crying out for help all the time and it isn't coming until it is too late. I think that once someone has cracked or lost it, it's a lot harder to pull them back on a line than if you get them before they snap."

Risk management for people living in the community is more likely to be successful when people receive a quick and effective response, should their mental state deteriorate. Uncertainty about whether such a response would be forthcoming was a cause of great concern to some service users and relatives. Problems or delays in getting treatment were mentioned in relation to seven service users. For example, one person waited eight months for their first psychiatric out-patient appointment. Another person had spent three days in a police cell waiting for a bed before a previous admission and some people talked about being turned away from psychiatric hospitals or accident and emergency departments in the past when asking for treatment. For example, one service user had gone to accident and emergency, the police were called and he had been threatened with obstruction and treated "terribly". One homeless man described turning up at hospital when "a bit depressed and a bit psychotic" and said:

"Some hospitals have refused me to see the doctors in the hospitals. They've refused me because I've turned up on the door saying that I'm ill and I've nowhere to live and things like that and they've just refused me – just, like, turned their back on me."

He rejected the need for services when admitted during the study and dropped out of contact with services as soon as possible. He may have been less likely to do so if his past experience had been better. Hospitals are not currently set up for self-referrals but it seems that the chance for collaborative work with this service user was missed.

One social worker said that it had taken two years for a service user with mental health and substance misuse problems to be accepted by the psychiatric services. He praised the consultant psychiatrist who offered the service user support, when he could have chosen not to. This problem reflects the national trend of people with a dual diagnosis often finding it difficult to access either mental health or substance misuse services. Recent guidance (DoH, 2002b) gives responsibility to mental health services to treat people with a dual diagnosis.

Delays were particularly worrying for the two service users who had a diagnosis of bipolar disorder (manic depression). They would realise that they were becoming unwell and seek help, but if it did not materialise within a matter of days, if not hours, they either refused services or had become a risk to others by that point. One service user talked about unsuccessfully asking for help on several occasions because a bed was not available. Before his last admission he had got a friend to take him to the local accident and emergency department in order to get into Middletown Hospital. The other service user had been 'signed off' from services before his last admission and it took considerable time and effort to reinvolve them. By admission he was in an extremely distressed and distressing state and had become a serious risk to a friend, which upset him greatly. He said:

"People don't realise it's not easy; you can't just ring up Middletown Hospital and say someone's ill, can you take them back? There seems to be this system which you've got to go through. And it is difficult actually to get someone in, especially a person like me who's, like, ill sort of every three years and not in the system all that long. It is difficult to get the assistance you need."

A few service users felt more confident that help would be made available in a crisis since systems had been established that would hopefully generate a quick response to any future difficulties. One service user talked about contacting ward staff at Valley Hospital and getting readmitted and another person was able to contact the hospital ward at weekends if he wanted.

Others were still concerned. For example, one person wondered if he would be able to get assistance quickly if, as had just happened, he became psychotic again after some years of being well and no longer any contact with mental health services.

Relatives' and friends' views of support

While all the service users lived independently of friends or relatives, the friends and relatives felt the impact of the service users' mental distress:

"You obviously get used to it, as best you can, but you are living like on a time bomb because you know the chances of it happening again are quite likely because it's happened a few times and it's an illness."

"And sometimes I think, 'Oh no, not again', as much as I loved him dearly but it's a big ordeal when you're going through it from my point of view."

Relatives and friends raised the following concerns:

- the person was given support quickly when their mental health was in crisis;
- services were not withdrawn too quickly.

Some also talked about:

- their distress where the service user rejected services or treatment that they thought helpful;
- having to provide high levels of support to a service user because the mental health services were not providing sufficient support themselves;
- not being listened to concerning the person's risk to relatives. One relative talked about how, on a previous admission, staff had not accepted his view that the service user was too much of a risk to family members to go home (which was where he lived at that point).

Despite his fears, the service user had been allowed to go home;

- an agreement to help a service user apply to college not materialising;
- a lack of understanding about the significance of family and independence in different cultures.

Friends and relatives expressed great concern about delays in getting support, as well as service users being discharged in the past with little or no support or accommodation. Indeed, one service user had ended up camping in his family's garden after a previous admission. However, he now had a social worker and psychiatrist putting much effort into finding him suitable accommodation. Doubts about whether a failsafe system could ever be set up were voiced by the following relative:

"But it's always going to happen on the odd occasion where it's a weekend, or the doctor's on holiday, or somebody's not there. It's always.... You know? So what do you do? Where do you go? Do I take him? I can't just admit him, you see. And sometimes there's not any beds."

Three relatives or friends talked about wanting a named person or organisation that they could go to for help rather than having to ring around various organisations to get a response. One person would have liked:

"… this sort of halfway house where you can go, and take your son, or whoever it might be, and say, 'Well, he's not very well'. You know? It would be nice if there was a place: it was between Middletown and a halfway house, if you like. When you were in distress everybody was welcome to go. You didn't have to sort of ring up here, ring there. You could go and say, 'We've got a bit of a problem. Can you help us?'."

He saw their role as:

"They could say, 'Well, yeah. I think we ought to get him to the doctor'. And they could help you, you know, because you're dealing with the ill person, aren't you, and you're not really right yourself are you? You're under stress so you want somebody to do the ringing around for you, don't you?"

Good practice suggestion: Relatives or friends of service users require information about how to access support for the service user. Protocols within community services (for example, GPs, the social services department, voluntary sector organisations and the mental health trust) could help ensure that there is a coordinated response to relatives or friends trying to get support for the service user.

Support not offered to service users

The following support was either not provided or provided only to some service users:

Responding to racist attacks

As described in Chapter 2, three of the four service users from minority ethnic groups had been attacked or abused because of their ethnic background.

Good practice suggestion: Action to tackle racism is needed at two levels.

- At an individual level, the implications of an attack or abuse for the service user need to be discussed, with the choice of doing so with a member of staff from a black or minority ethnic group. Where such a member of staff does not exist, an advocate from a black or minority ethnic group or an organisation supporting victims of racism should be involved.
- At an institutional level, the safety of service users from black or minority ethnic groups, while in hospital, needs to be considered and where attacks take place, an investigation of whether they have a racial element is needed.

One service user had been housed in an area characterised by tension between different minority ethnic groups and both he and a relative had been attacked and threatened. The only drop-in centre was primarily for members of the same minority ethnic group that had attacked him and which he did not want to attend.

Good practice suggestion: Greater sensitivity to the needs of people from different minority ethnic groups will help avoid a 'one size fits all' approach.

Cultural issues

Differences in cultural expectations about work, independence and family were not always clearly understood between service users, families and mental health staff. One relative said that the service user had 'become more English cultured' and felt that he no longer gave his family the same respect.

One social worker talked about trying unsuccessfully to find a group for young men from the same minority ethnic background. A young people's project had been rejected because it involved a camping trip, something not part of his cultural norms. The worker also said:

"The concern [is] around that he's from an ethnic minority and ensuring that these things [that is, his culture] are taken on board rather than ignored by the mental health services. I think that's still an on-going issue. But it probably isn't reflected in the services that he's getting."

Another issue was the assumption of common interests purely on the basis of colour. One man was referred to a centre for people from one minority ethnic group with whom he had nothing in common and where tensions between the two groups had spilled over into violence, including violence towards himself and a family member.

The issue of respecting other culture's ways of responding to mental distress was also important. Two service users had consulted spiritual healers and one worker described this as going to a 'magic doctor'.

The following requirements relate to staff:

i) training to counter institutional racism was needed for all workers, for example race equality training, cultural awareness and a review of strategies;
ii) internalised racism.

Staff from minority ethnic groups working in institutions that are racist may internalise that racism. One worker said he had never seen any racism towards service users whereas in relation to a service user, another worker said:

"But I think something's happened along the way where he feels very worthless ... and he's black as well, I mean in my experience, black men don't fare particularly well in the mental health system."

Support for refugees and asylum seekers

The service user who had fled his war-torn country had not been put in touch with support agencies for refugees or asylum seekers, nor was he receiving any counselling for the effects of trauma.

Support for children

No attention was given to the mental health of the young family members of service users in this study. However, workers were aware of this as an issue and there were plans for one child whose parent had long-term mental health problems to get psychological help. The lack of attention to the needs of children where their parent has mental health difficulties is an issue of national concern (Youngminds website). Research also suggests problems between mental health and childcare professionals working together effectively to meet needs (Hetherington et al, 2002).

Childcare was also needed for parents who brought their young family with them on visits to the service user or to meetings with professionals.

Advocacy

It was surprising that advocacy was not used more, particularly for those service users who found it difficult to express their views or were unhappy with services offered.

Good practice suggestion: All service users require information about:

- local advocacy services;
- the range of therapies available within the NHS (so that they can make an informed choice about what support they want to be referred for).

Therapeutic input

Some people were offered psychological help for hearing voices, childhood abuse or racial discrimination. However, there were other service users who may have equally benefited but were not offered this or other support such as family therapy. A few service users said that they would have liked some therapeutic input, for example examining underlying reasons for their distress:

"There's always a reason why someone gets an illness. And there's so many schools of thought with illness that, like, genetic – another theory's imbalance in the brain. But I think a lot of the medical profession, now, don't really want to find out why. They just know you've got an illness and they treat it with drugs instead of a real deep counselling."

Substance abuse

While workers discussed problematic substance misuse with service users, only two service users were receiving specialist help. A sharing of expertise between mental health and substance misuse workers may have been helpful, but one difficulty was in getting local substance misuse services to accept a service user experiencing psychosis.

Anger management

Although many of the service users could be potentially threatening towards other people or property when experiencing psychosis, no one had been offered any specialist anger management programme.

Relapse prevention

In terms of relapse prevention, no one was involved in self-help or self-management groups provided by the Hearing Voices Network or the Manic Depression Fellowship. A few service users were involved in plans for relapse prevention or had been given strategies to assist them to stay well while others, who could equally have benefited from this approach, were not.

Good practice suggestions:

- Every service user should have a document about what to do should their mental condition or behaviour deteriorate, that is, a relapse plan as well as what to do in a crisis. (This is now government policy.)
- Copies should only be given to involved friends or relatives with service user agreement unless there are sufficiently serious risks to justify breaching confidentiality.
- Service users should be informed about self-management strategies developed by groups such as the Hearing Voices Network or the Manic Depression Fellowship.

However, service user involvement in relapse prevention depends on agreement that certain behaviours are of concern and, as has already been discussed in Chapter 4, this was not always present. For example, one man thought that a worker was trying to harm him. It proved impossible to discuss relapse prevention strategies since he did not agree that these thoughts were a sign that he was becoming unwell or a potential risk to others.

Quality of life

When service users were asked what would improve their quality of life, they mentioned aspirations common to all of us, such as having a long-term relationship, having a holiday, being an active member of the community, living in a better environment or doing some travelling.

Some service users' wish to find work, go to college or university or follow up creative interests such as art classes were supported and indeed encouraged. However, others had interests that they wanted to pursue that professionals were unaware of. For example, one man was interested in art and carpentry, another wanted to go horse riding and another person wanted a holiday since he had not had one for 10 years.

Good practice suggestion: There needs to be systematic discussion with individual service users of their skills, abilities and interests so that plans can be made to support or develop them.

Several service users said that they wanted to be put something back into their community:

"Say, in five years, I'd like to see myself working, paying my own rent and supporting my children. Yeah, just being a functioning, symbiotic member of society. I'd really like that. I could really contribute."

Two service users mentioned that they would like to engage in exercise but that they did not have the funds to do this, whereas none of their community-based workers mentioned this.

Relationships

"Yeah, I can talk to Dr X. I really like her. I really feel that she understands me and I do feel that she's on my side."

Service users' views about staff and their helpfulness towards them varied and characteristics that were valued included:

- a doctor "who actually listens to me";
- staff who listened to a service user's desire to cut herself, asked her not to do it that day "and it doesn't take away my right to do it";
- staff who were happy to spend time talking with the service user, rather than, as one service user said, telling him to go away five minutes later.

However, a small number of staff were considered patronising (mainly consultant psychiatrists), "just doing their job" or seen as caring about the service user but trying to force unwanted services on the person.

"They're saying, 'We care about you' or 'We're keeping you in here for your own protection'.... They're not keeping me in here for my own protection, they're just saying they care about me. Right? Then why don't they listen to me when I say that I'm ready to do things?"

All the workers talked about the importance of a good relationship between themselves and the service user in averting crises and managing risk. Many examples were given of the influence this made to a service user's willingness to accept services. One worker said that because a service user enjoyed an activity group, he was more likely to go to psychiatric review appointments and to contact the hospital out of hours if concerned about his mental state.

Neither professionals, nor their managers, had developed a means of systematically evaluating how service users experienced the support offered and whether they found professionals effective and helpful.

Good practice suggestion: Since a good working relationship between a service user and professionals is seen as key:

a) Professionals and their managers need to develop methods to evaluate how helpful service users find services provided as well as their views about the professionals involved in their lives.
b) A choice of changing the worker should be made available where service users feel that there is little or no rapport between themselves and their worker. (This may demand more flexibility than is available, for example where a consultant psychiatrist covers a wide geographical area).
c) People using mental health services on a long-term basis should not routinely be seen by trainee doctors working on a six-monthly rotation.

Communication

Workers saw effective communication between themselves as crucial in managing risk. There were many examples of the care coordinators' close contact with everyone involved with the service user. However, there were also examples where workers in the voluntary sector or a drop-in service did not receive enough information, for example after discharge from hospital.

Effective communication between service users, relatives or friends and professionals is clearly crucial in terms of effective support and risk management. As already mentioned, some service users found it relatively easy to express their views about services and support. Others did not, including some whose dissatisfaction with services was not known by professionals.

Some staff were more prepared than others to find language and sign language interpreters for interviews with the relatives of service users. In this research, we used a local language interpretation service. However, we found the following problems with some interpreters: not translating the exact words of interviewees, summarising their answers, the interpreter interjecting their own opinion or adding information gained from interpreting for the relatives in other settings, for example at a care plan meeting.

Good practice suggestions:

- Systems need to be set up to ensure that there is full communication of information with everyone involved with the service user, given the usual safeguards about confidentiality. Attention to the need for interpreters, including British Sign Language interpreters, as well as considering ways of involving more fully people who find it difficult to express their views, is required.
- Interpreter training in confidentiality, accuracy (including not summarising what people say) and specialist knowledge of mental health is needed.

Continuity of care

Continuity of care allows relationships to develop and several workers mentioned that knowing a service user over time stopped them over-reacting:

"I see some of the younger nurses getting really frightened and saying, 'Oh, my God! Call the team.' And all these young, eager nurses appear and have some physical contact and he doesn't need it. You just go along and say, 'Hello X. How you doing? Have a cigarette. Let's go for a walk, it's nice weather. Are you all right?' If one of the nurses that knows him can remove him from the situation the whole thing just calms right down."

Good practice suggestion: Information about successful ways of calming individual service users who become agitated or angry should be placed in a prominent place within care records. The service user's views about what helps in such situations should be included.

Trust and collaborative relationships take time to build but when service users moved they often became involved with a different community mental health team. Two problems were associated with this: delays in seeing a new worker and the service user's unwillingness to engage with a new team when previously happy about involvement. One ward manager said that there needed to be a stronger focus on continuity of care as, in her experience, people became lost to services and risk assessments were not handed over, thereby increasing risk for everyone. After discharge, several service users were moving to new teams because of moving house (after the standard hand-over period of six months) which raises the possibility of similar problems occurring.

Several service users were dissatisfied with frequent changes of doctor, some being seen by a different doctor virtually every time they went to an out-patient appointment:

"Just as you're getting somewhere with a psychiatrist, then they're off.... Like I said, you loose the whole incentive of what you had before, of getting somewhere and working on the good work, and then that person's gone. And the next consultant ... they'd have a different approach to the way they deal with it. So you do lose a lot of progress with the changes on a regular basis.... Because every doctor I've known has been different. They've all got their different views and they've all got ways of dealing with an individual person."

This comment illustrates not only the difficulty of having to get to know new staff and adjust to their ways of doing things, but also the lack of power that service users have over what support is offered, as well as the shortage of psychiatrists.

Good practice examples:

- One social worker continued to see a service user after he moved due to concern that the new team would not accept him because of their long waiting list and tight eligibility criteria.
- A hospital keyworker undertaking therapy, who only saw hospital in-patients, continued to see one service user after discharge. He thought that the person already had enough changes to adjust to, since he was moving into new accommodation and his consultant psychiatrist, with whom he had a good relationship, was leaving.

Good practice questions:

1. How can established plans agreed between the service user and doctor, or care coordinator, be respected when there are staff changes?
2. How can systems be set up to access help quickly for people in crisis who have not had recent contact with mental health services?

Ethical dilemmas

Although the majority of professionals said that they did not have any ethical dilemmas when working with the service users, a few mentioned the following:

Confidentiality

Some professionals said that there was a tension between communicating with relatives and maintaining confidentiality, for example, when relatives were being asked by service users for money which they suspected was to buy street drugs:

"I don't want to exclude them from his care but, at the same time, I don't want to divulge too much about … particularly in terms of my being fairly suspicious about his use of drugs. So without sort of explicitly saying that, I suggested that if he needed food and cigarettes and that if he wanted money off them then perhaps they could give some food and some cigarettes

to him – give that to him as a support. And that would be a way of ensuring that if he was taking drugs that he wouldn't be spending their money on that. So … an ethical balancing act really!"

Another worker's comments showed that he thought that patient confidentiality was being sacrificed in favour of communication with families:

"And I think there is that issue: we're working, now, very much in partnership with families and carers and wanting them to be involved, which is good, but I think there's always a danger that we swing a bit too far and, you know, confidentiality slips a bit."

Relatives and friends generally understood that staff could not breach confidentiality, although the following comment suggests some frustration about this as well as professionals trying to strike a balance between two competing priorities – providing information and maintaining confidentiality:

"You know, even talking with the nurse, you know, I could say, 'How is he? You know, what's he doing?' And he said, 'Well, I can't really tell you that'. And I say, 'Well, do I have to ask a hundred and one questions? Will you give me the right answer? You know, if I ask the question, you can answer it, but you can't actually tell me?' And they go, 'Yes'."

Even where a service user agreed to a worker speaking to relatives, deciding how much information the service user would think acceptable was a source of tension:

"I don't think his sister knows perhaps a tenth of what he gets up to really. And that's an area that I've got to be very careful with him about because I do have knowledge of that. But that's still confidential to X. Even though I've got his consent to talk to them, there are limits towards that. If I sort of said to them, 'Oh, X's taking drugs all the time and that's where all his money's going' and all this sort of thing, then that would be too much of a breach of confidentiality. I wouldn't enter into that."

Confidentiality can be breached where the person is considered to be a sufficiently high risk to themselves or other people. The stage at which this should happen was problematic for one worker who gave the example of a relative asking, 'Is he breaking down? Is he becoming unwell again?'.

> Good practice suggestion: Protocols about confidentiality should be individualised and negotiated between the service user, any relatives or carers and the mental health professionals. They should include an agreement about the circumstances under which confidentiality could be breached where a service user does not want contact between professionals and relatives or carers.

Unease about drug misuse

A few staff working in the statutory sector (that is, the trust or the social services department) were uneasy about the service user taking illegal drugs since they felt that it compromised their position.

Personal responsibility

Several people would have been charged with a criminal offence if they had not been admitted to hospital and some professionals mentioned the ethical dilemma of how much responsibility the service user should bear when violent towards others:

> "You know, he's detained under the Mental Health Act and, yet, there are a lot of people who feel that he should be responsible if he goes to housing and assaults somebody or tries to assault somebody, that he should be charged. And yet he's under the Mental Health Act so is that going to get him off of everything?"

In an article about risk, we have suggested the following (Langan and Lindow, 2000, p 14):

> A professional also needs to consider how far any possible dangerousness is part of ordinary levels of dangerousness in our society. For example it is ethical to treat domestic violence or a breach of the peace on a Saturday night, as symptoms of mental illness rather than as illegal behaviour? Does this sometimes prevent the person from taking responsibility for their own behaviour?

Medication

Since the majority of workers thought that the person's use of medication was beneficial (as discussed in Chapter 6), enforcing medication was an ethical dilemma for only a few workers. Several housing support workers mentioned the moral dilemma of whether to support or dissuade a service user who did not want to take medication. As previously mentioned, one nurse saw 'persuading' people to stay on medication for the rest of their lives as an ethical dilemma.

Money

One social worker restricted a service user's access to his own money. She described the service user as someone who used all his benefit on drugs and then aggressively threatened others for money. The worker concerned saw controlling access to money as an ethical dilemma but felt that everyone's best interests were served by doing this.

One social worker felt uneasy about helping one service user complete forms for Disability Living Allowance, when he was convinced that the person would use the benefit to buy street drugs.

Summary

This chapter has shown that plans to manage risk were generally done on an informal basis as part of the care planning process. Service users were not always clearly informed that risk management was included within that process. Service users' ability to influence the outcomes was determined by a number of factors: how articulate and determined they were to be involved (since advocates were not used), how serious their risk behaviour had been (and therefore how much public protection took precedence) and how much they knew about available services. However, ultimately the care plan was very much within the gift of the professional, albeit that many professionals we spoke with worked hard to develop a plan that

the service user would find acceptable. Delays
in support were a great cause of concern to
service users and relatives and, on the basis of
both what some service users said and our
knowledge of the range of possible services,
some support needs were not being met. We
recommend the implementation of an
information strategy to inform people about what
services are available, plus greater use of
advocacy services to increase the chances of
people receiving services that they want. We
also recommend that systematic means be found
to establish service users' views about the
support given.

6

Medication and housing issues

In this chapter we discuss:

- medication becoming part of some service users' psychosis;
- staff attitudes towards medication;
- service users' views about medication;
- substance misuse and medication;
- service users' reasons for not wanting to take medication;
- harmful side-effects as a consequence of taking medication;
- insecurity in accommodation;
- supported housing.

Medication

Encouraging a person to take medication, especially someone considered to pose a potential risk to others, is almost invariably the cornerstone of any risk management strategy. Yet it is often a source of dispute and disagreement between service users and professionals.

The Draft Mental Health Bill (DoH, 2002) gives medication even more of a central role so that it will become more difficult for people living in the community to refuse medication thought necessary by professionals. A popular view is that if only the person took their medication, risk would be eliminated or significantly reduced. Yet in their analysis of a number of homicide inquiry reports, Parker and McCulloch (1999) found that the following factors, in their order of importance, all preceded non-compliance with medication as significant factors involved in homicides by people with a diagnosis of mental illness:

- poor risk management;
- communication problems;
- inadequate care planning;
- lack of inter-agency working;
- administrative and procedural failures;

- lack of suitable accommodation;
- poor resources;
- substance misuse.

The proposed legislation addresses 'non-compliance' by providing for compulsory medication while not guaranteeing to users services that evidence suggests would have much more effect in reducing rare dangers. Only a few workers commented on the proposals in the White Paper *Reform of the Mental Health Act 1983* (DoH, 1999b) to force service users to take medication while living in the community. However, those that did comment were, with one exception, unhappy about the proposals. Reasons centred on the practical difficulties with implementation and the harm they would cause to relationships with service users in terms of reducing trust and collaboration as well as increasing the likelihood of their disengagment from services:

"So, in some ways, for reasons which are perfectly sound about civil liberties in life, we are in a position where we don't have all the answers, I suppose really, to managing risk. Obviously, given a different structure, we might be able to manage the risk more actively and more directly. But whether we would actually want that, in terms of what it would mean to the way the service worked and what that would do to people's actual rights to choose, I think would be very difficult."

Medication becoming part of some service users' psychosis

One area of media and public misunderstanding is about cause and effect in the use of medication. The general assumption that not taking medication always leads to relapse was not borne out in this study. While many staff spoke about service users' decisions not to take their medication as the *cause* of a relapse, some staff and service users described the opposite situation. That is, medication was being taken but did not prevent a relapse. Stress caused a relapse and the relapse may have contributed to the person stopping their medication:

"He does [take medication] until there is some trigger and he's stressed and then, the next step in how things go for him will be he'll start to feel that the medication is poison and he shouldn't take it."

Staff attitudes towards medication

Ensuring 'compliance' with medication was seen by virtually all professionals as crucially important in managing risk. In cases where negotiation was unsuccessful, coercion more accurately described the process. Many said that they had seen dramatic improvements in mental health due to medication. Relatives also tended to agree with the view that medication is always beneficial. However, five workers expressed concern about medication's predominance in care plans. One nurse said that he believed in 'anti-psychotics' in an acute episode, but saw recommending to the service user that they took neuroleptic drugs for the rest of their life as an ethical dilemma:

"Do we really want people on Section Three for the rest of their lives having Depots [injections]? It's not practical and I wonder about its efficacy."

It was clear that staff spent considerable amounts of time trying to find medication that was effective and that did not have too many side-effects, so that many of the service users were regularly trying out new or additional medication. One social worker said:

"You know, you are left wondering how advanced we are in our treatment in helping people with, you know, very severe psychotic illnesses.... Nothing seems to shift his pattern of thinking, that you would call a psychotic illness or thought disturbance of some sort. And I think it's there all the time, virtually. And treatment allows him to cope with it but it doesn't get rid of it."

Service users' views about medication

Medication was an important issue for all the service users and everyone was receiving medication at the first interview. Sixteen service users had 'anti-psychotic' and/or 'mood-stabilising' medication on a long-term basis, with several of this latter group also taking 'anti-depressants'. Some were prescribed other drugs to help control side effects. The final service user was prescribed 'anti-depressants' only. We use inverted commas here because although many people were helped by medication, both psychosis and depression continued to be a feature of several people's lives. The naming of these groups of drugs may imply greater efficacy than they actually have. While all staff viewed medication as beneficial, some saw 'anti-psychotic' medication as only partially so, even for some people on maximum doses.

All but one service user had 'accepted' medication in hospital, possibly knowing that refusal could have led to the Mental Health Act being used to ensure compliance. The one service user who refused 'anti-psychotic' medication was forcibly injected, which he described as "degrading". At the second interview phase, two service users had moved out of hospital under Section (in order to ensure 'compliance' with medication) and a third service user was spending more time in hospital than at home with 'non-compliance' one reason for this. Another two people had refused medication, and a third who had rejected psychiatric services, was not thought to be taking any. Another service user, who moved out of hospital under Section to ensure 'compliance' with medication, swore that he would stop it as soon as he could. His desire to be free from medication led to him feeling frustrated that workers did not understand his point of view and that they were trying to control him. His doctor was giving what he considered to be the lowest possible dose but this was not what the service user wanted. There is clearly a tension here for staff between persuasion (which can ultimately led to disengagement) and allowing a service user to make what they feel is an unwise choice.

Of the other service users, some were now on medication which they found helpful:

"I've got to watch out. I don't want to hurt anyone else and I don't want to get hurt myself. I want to live my life quietly – in peace and quiet. There's a lot in life for me with the help of Depixol and the health service people."

Another service user had agreed to take the Depot injections (recommended by professionals where 'compliance' is an issue):

"All the time I was at the day hospital they always used to say would I like to try Depot. I always felt safer just taking the pills because I could regulate it. But after this last thing where I just exploded, sort of thing, and did something very stupid, the Depot's the perfect thing for me, yeah."

Others were ambivalent or 'non-compliant' (as described by some staff) about taking medication at some point during their cycle of mental health crisis and stability. No service user suggested that staff were 'non-compliant' with their wishes in this or any other context: a reflection of the differences between them in terms of position and power. Where service users disagreed with the need for medication, staff often said that the service user lacked 'insight'. However, some workers showed sensitivity towards the issue:

"Ambivalence about the medication is normal rather than kind of pathological, so I'm not saying, by any token idea, that it's part of a lack of insight.... You know, it's quite a normal.... Tell *me* to take medication every day. 'No' is the answer!"

The level of ambivalence about medication, even among those taking it, raises questions about how likely it was that 'compliance' would be maintained.

Another reason given for ambivalence was the enforced or high dosages of medication administered to some service users while in hospital (not necessarily during their most recent admission). This experience, often their first of medication, remained part of their perception of medication. Few staff mentioned this possible negative effect on service users' willingness to take prescribed drugs:

"They put me on a very high dose of medication, which almost killed me. And they didn't really think nothing of it. They were telling me I was crazy if I was saying

they were trying to kill me. They said they were trying to help me but they nearly killed me with too much medication."

These fears echo the continuing controversy over the extent to which psychiatric medication is implicated in 'sudden unexplained deaths'. The National Confidential Inquiry into Suicide and Homicide has expanded its remit to consider nationally the risks factors associated with sudden unexplained deaths in psychiatric hospitals (Appleby et al, 2000).

Substance misuse and medication

It was striking that the service users most happily taking medication were those with a dual diagnosis, of whom six were considered to use psychiatric medication 'addictively'. These service users, knowledgeable about the effects of medication, would ask for prescribed drugs with effects that mirrored those found in street drugs or alcohol. One man was described as 'loving medication' by a worker who said that 'he used it almost like an illicit substance'. One service user said:

"You see, benzodiazepines are on offer here as well. And that's the ones that everyone likes to take because they chill you out. Umm. Warmed out. Nice feeling. Very calm. Very at peace.... The only problem is that they're addictive so the doctors don't like to give you them very much."

Staff did not see enthusiasm for medication as unproblematic. One worker was concerned that a high dosage might harm one service user in the long term. One nurse described giving another person benzodiazepines, although he no longer felt that they were clinically necessary and the service user had already been taking them for longer than three weeks (the point at which it is possible to become addicted to them). However, the service user was keen to have them. Mainly staff were pleased when the person willingly took medication:

"If that's because he feels that the medication is a bit of a downer and, you know, it's on tap and it's cheaper than smack, then, if that's his reason for taking it, then so be it. I'd rather he took it for that reason than didn't take it at all."

The inability of some service users taking street drugs (such as amphetamines or cannabis) to take medication regularly concerned staff. Service users may have been willing but were considered too disorganised to attend out-patients appointments to review medication and be given a prescription.

Service users' reasons for not wanting to take medication

- *Not 'mentally ill':* three service users did not agree that they had a 'mental illness' and so trying to persuade them to take medication which may have unwelcome side-effects becomes even more problematic.

- *Not wanting to take medication when well:* some service users accepted their diagnosis, but not that they should take medication. One man told of his unsuccessful attempt to stop taking medication. Having been well for some time, he had decided to reduce his medication by half and then decided to come off all medication. This, in his view, had led to him becoming seriously psychotic and, for the first time, to be considered a potential risk to other people (this resulted in a hospital admission which made him think that he would have to stay on medication for the foreseeable future):

  "I was a damn fool because I burnt my bridges by doing that. I should have come down by a quarter and also made sure that there were plenty of back-up tranquillisers in the cupboard should I feel a bit raw."

He also said that he should have ensured staff support since one aspect of his experience coming off the medication was that "all the sides of yourself that aren't being suppressed [by the drugs], start coming back", so that he was trying to deal with feelings pre-dating him taking medication.

- *Fears about dependency on medication:* a few service users talked about not wanting to be dependent on medication. One man talked about wanting to "get hold of his life" and

"feel free". This does not seem an unreasonable stance given society's views on drug dependence, echoed forcefully by the mental health system's taking drug dependence into its cohort of 'mental illnesses'.

- *Medication being ineffective:* service users talked about the limits of medication and giving them up because they did not work. One service user mentioned knowing people who became unwell even when taking medication. For the above reasons, clinical insistence on continuous medication to prevent relapse was less than convincing to some.

- *The harmfulness of medication:* another service user felt damaged by injections that he did not want and frustrated that mental health staff did not acknowledge how he felt about the injury that he felt was being done to him:

  "And I say to the doctors, 'If by any chance there is another life, I'll have you all back. I'll put an injection into your legs and see how you like it'. It's not nice at all. No, not at all."

However, his psychiatrist seemed unaware of the strength of his views:

  "He actually seems reasonably comfortable on it. I mean, medication has not been a big issue for him as far as I'm aware. Well, no more of an issue for him than it is for anybody I suppose. No, generally, he's pretty, you know, reasonably compliant. He's never sort of resisted medication."

Harmful side-effects as a consequence of taking medication

All the service users taking 'anti-psychotic' medication (16) either had current or past experience of side-effects, with 14 service users telling us about this themselves. Family, friends or staff members described side-effects for the other two service users. Many people were taking more than one drug plus medication to control unwanted side-effects. The fact that some side-effects were controlled in this way did not stop their concern about the toxic nature of their drugs.

Many staff understood service users' reports of side-effects and worked with them to try to find a tolerable drug. One community psychiatric nurse thought that: "the reason why most of my clients refuse the medication is their sedative effects". (Even the newer 'anti-psychotic' drugs had their problems because they have to be taken regularly and blood tests need to be carried out because they can have dangerous and possibly fatal side-effects.)

Some service users continued to take medication despite side-effects. For others this was a major issue and staff were concerned that about whether this would cause them to stop the medication in the future. Staff generally thought that medication was 'the lesser of two evils', but for some service users the side-effects were so distressing and debilitating that medication became the greater evil.

Only two members of staff mentioned systematic monitoring for side-effects and a few service users talked to us about side-effects that workers were unaware of.

Good practice suggestion: All service users should be asked regularly about the presence of any side-effects and this information should be recorded.

Mental effects

One subtle aspect of how people described their side-effects illustrates that they feel that their core sense of self is destroyed by taking anti-psychotic medication:

"It's like a breeze-block being lowered on your head and you can't, like, be yourself."

"You feel a little bit plasticated, sort of thing.... Sort of like a cardboard cut-out of a person."

Talking about wanting to stop taking the medication when well, one service user said:

"It was just that I wanted to set my soul free."

This person's relative said something similar:

"You know, they dampen his being, as it were."

Another relative also remarked on this in the context of the service user not being able to 'show grief or real reality' because of the medication.

For some service users, a change of medication had improved matters, while others experienced psychological effects such as nightmares (including flashbacks during the day), strange thoughts, an inability to think and hearing voices due to medication. However, staff sometimes could not accept what service users told them, that the quality of life on medication was not acceptable to them as a permanent solution. Some did not seem to register the core-person-changing nature of the experience of psychiatric drugs. One worker commented: "It doesn't have to affect his life, you know, he can do everything he wants to do on it", about someone who was extremely ambivalent about medication, with good cause, due to its psychological effects.

Physical effects

Two service users experienced particularly serious physical side-effects during the study. One had a catheter for four months due to urinary retention probably caused, according to the psychiatrist, by nerve damage to his bladder from Depot injections. Another service user had taken extra doses of medication when unwell and had ended up in casualty as a medical emergency with severe eye problems.

Other physical side-effects mentioned by service users were nausea, thirst, continual pains in joints, "crippling stiffness and juddering", continual leg shaking, lack of coordination, a stiff face, muscle spasms, diarrhoea, speech impairment and "a weird kind of tiredness". Fitness levels were affected by limb stiffness or the sedative effects of medication. Weight gain, with its effects on self-image, also affected some. Medication exacerbated the pain one service user experienced from a physical condition. Some were also concerned about the long-term effects on their physical health:

"'Cos mental health drugs are very sort of absorbent. Do you know what I mean? They do absorb in the body quite a lot and it can, in time, cause a lot of problems if you're on medication for years."

Another serious side-effect of old-style 'anti-psychotic' medication, not mentioned by service users, but mentioned by staff in relation to three people, was interference with sexual functioning. One ward keyworker said:

"Sexual dysfunction is a big one. With the young blokes, you get raised prolactin levels, which either makes it difficult to get an erection or difficult to actually climax once you've got an erection.... Every young bloke's aim who I've ever worked with has been to get a nice girlfriend and keep a nice girlfriend. If you've got a sexual dysfunction due to your medication then you're going to choose to keep going with your medication or choose to jack it in."

This worker was among those in favour of moving people on to newer 'atypical' medication, sold by pharmaceutical companies as having fewer side-effects. However, this was not always possible with this group of service users, either because of their refusal to change their medication or because the newer drugs were not available in the form of injections which can be more easily monitored by staff.

Differences of opinion over side-effects

In most, but not all cases, staff accepted the service user's views about side-effects. One service user was thought to keep hospital staff interested in him by complaining of side-effects 'out of the blue' whereas the service user said, "I've always got pains in my legs all the time". The difficulty for professionals of disentangling the side-effects of prescribed medication from those of 'coming down' after a period of taking street drugs such as amphetamines was also mentioned.

Good practice examples:

Many of the following examples may be routine in some services, but impressed the researchers as taking extra time and trouble.

Trying various drugs
• Some service users felt that they had exercised some choice and that their viewpoint was respected.
• Many clinical staff spent time and energy trying to find medication that was effective or did not have unwelcome or dangerous side-effects.
• One service user had used his GP to persuade a psychiatrist that he could continue the drug he felt suited him, rather than change to another that the psychiatrist felt had fewer side-effects. However, it was not always possible for psychiatrists to find a drug combination without serious side-effects.

Negotiation
• Some service users reported that they had been 'allowed' to change medication.
• Staff described having 'allowed' service users to take more medication on demand than they might have recommended but which the service user felt was needed.

Flexibility
• In providing medication via the community psychiatric nurse despite the person not seeing their psychiatrist or taking medication regularly.
• Adopting a relatively relaxed attitude to street drugs, especially cannabis, when used as self-medication.
• Giving smaller and more frequent doses of a Depot injection that, when given in the normal doseage, had exacerbated the pain a service user experienced from a physical condition.

Seeing someone through serious physical illness
• Both his residential placement and the mental health services had supported one service user through tests and treatment for a life-threatening illness. He had been readmitted to psychiatric hospital to have nursing care for his physical health problems. From the point of view of medication, his weight had been carefully monitored and the dosages adjusted according to loss and subsequently weight gain.

Offering an advocate
- One professional gave contact details of an advocacy service to a service user who felt that his views about medication were not given sufficient weight.

Systematically monitoring side-effects
- While this was done in a minority of cases, its use could be extremely helpful to service users for staff to systematically monitor for and record potentially harmful side-effects.

Not always increasing medication levels/trying out alternative strategies
- One member of staff, who described a service user's frightening and aggressive behaviour on the ward, illustrated the possibility of alternative action:

> "It's easy to see him and then think, 'Oh, my God! Lots of medication', which he does need. But it's easy to think, 'Why don't we get a team together and sit on him and restrain him [control restraint] and then give him lots of medication?'. When, in fact, you just actually wander up to him and say, 'You're frightening people. Do you want a cigarette? Let's go for a walk'. It's better to walk him round the block three times than it is to stick a needle in him."

Information about medication
- A few service users had been provided with good information about their medication and any side-effects.
- A psychiatrist had written to a pharmaceutical company to clarify a point that the service user had raised and had given the information to the service user.

We did not find any examples of the following but suggest it as good practice:

- Discussing the effect on the person's self-identity of taking medication.

The term 'compliance' is being replaced within healthcare with that of 'concordance', which is a negotiated agreement about treatment between clinician and health service user. Whether or not that becomes a reality in mental healthcare remains to be seen. We end the discussion of medication with a recommendation from a service user with many years of experience of psychiatric medication:

> "So, really, for people who have been on anti-psychotic tranquillisers a long time, there needs to be provision. If the Department of Health – the government – could be so generous, there needs to be provision for some kind of centres where people can go for drying out. They don't currently have this at the moment but it's been talked about before. I would like that idea to be looked at again because I still think that if I'd been able to get off the [major tranquilliser] a long, long time ago, I might have experienced years of life without it by now. But because I've been on it all the time, because all my attempts to get off it have just been short, sharp and immediately straight off the damn stuff, then, of course, every last time I've been thrown back into psychosis and back into the mental hospital."

Housing

> "You know, I just want to get out and work, get my own flat and sort my life out again."

Housing is vital to securing someone's quality of life and when looking at housing issues in this study the two most noticeable aspects were:

- the current and past insecurity of accommodation experienced by service users;
- disagreement between service users and professionals about the value of supported housing.

Insecurity in accommodation

Only seven service users lived in the same place throughout the study. Six people lived in independent housing and one in supported housing. The other 10 people were homeless either at or during admission. Four people lost tenancies due to neglect and/or concerns about risk to, or conflict with, neighbours about noise, unpredictable behaviour, assaults or serious threats. Not every service user agreed with these assessments of their situation and two had been on the receiving end of harassment. But where neighbours had complained to the police and/or the housing manager, action had been taken leading to homelessness or giving up a tenancy for all but one of the people involved in these conflicts. One man was only notified that he was being evicted from social housing when he had his bags packed ready to go home from hospital.

Three people effectively became homeless because they refused to return to their supported housing, in two cases because of fears for their own safety. One person, while not technically homeless, was not being allowed to return home by his consultant due to concerns about risk. Another person had been in a hostel for homeless people before admission and was thought to need more support after discharge than it could provide.

The last homeless service user was the only person that professionals agreed from the outset should be helped to gain independent housing so that she could provide a home for herself and her children after discharge. She had involved a legal advocate at her care planning meeting and insisted on housing within the area where she had good support networks despite resistance from the housing department. This seemed entirely understandable and as she said herself:

"I'm not in a position to reform social networks or build social networks for my children – I'm not in a well enough state to do that."

While the medical staff fully supported her stance, another worker thought otherwise:

"She'd been offered several properties but refused them because she was really rigid and wouldn't move out of the area."

Supported housing

"I don't want to be in X any longer because they talk down to you as if you're a little child, basically. At the end of the day, they nose into your business."

Supported housing was seen by professionals as an important element in minimising risk. They saw supported housing as ideal for nine of the 10 homeless service users, while service users tended to want their own home with a secure tenancy. (The one person in supported housing

among the group whose accommodation stayed unchanged throughout the study had to move back there after discharge as he was under Section. However, he wanted his own flat).

Supported housing was agreed to readily by only a small number of service users. It had clear benefits for one person who lived in a scheme that gave him a secure tenancy in a self-contained flat (after a trial period), but with on-site staff and shared facilities if tenants wanted to use them. This was acceptable to the service user and had a different ethos from most mental health supported housing. The service user was not interested in relating to fellow tenants beyond saying 'hello' but liked the non-mental health staff and was still visited by his community psychiatric nurse The second person moved to new supported accommodation after refusing to return to his previous placement because of fears about aggression from other residents. He did not want independent housing and was happy to accept high levels of support.

None of the remaining service users wanted to go into supported housing. Where it had been tried before and failed, staff did not enforce it. One worker commented that making someone live somewhere against their wishes could lead to them disengaging from services as well as lead to the accommodation failing:

"If you go against what somebody wants and you work really hard to get them into an environment where *you* think they'd be better, one thing is that you're going against what that person's telling you and, are they actually going to comply with that environment? I mean, that's why the previous thing failed because he didn't like it there."

Two people moved into supported housing with a Section used to enforce this. One person was not being allowed to return home because of concerns about his risk to others and the other person's request for independent housing was not accepted.

"The staff team have taken very much the view that, 'If you go ahead and you can do that, you do that, but we're not going to support you in looking for independent accommodation. But we will help you in looking for a more supported area'."

In both cases, supported housing had never been tried before and this may have been one reason why it was enforced.

> Good practice example: One service user effectively ruined any chance of being offered supported housing by telling the providers that he had no intention of curbing his use of street drugs. As one worker said:
>
> > "Most supported housing projects are looking for a commitment from people to want to tackle their drug problems."
>
> The service user therefore moved into independent housing. Despite staff pessimism about the outcome, high levels of support were offered and accepted, that is, a community care worker for practical issues concerning accommodation, regular visits from a community psychiatric nurse and day hospital groups that the service user found useful and enjoyable. Workers were delighted with this man's progress, which was beyond their expectations.

Another issue that arose concerned levels of support. One service user, who also wanted his own flat, would have been prepared to accept supported housing but with minimal levels of support. However, since he was considered a high risk to others:

> "The less supported projects, that X would go for, are the ones that will never take him. And the ones that have 24-hour support may consider him but X is never going to consider them."

Supported housing may also carry risks. Service users' reasons for not wanting to live in supported housing were fear of fellow residents, being treated like a child and the difficulty of living in close proximity with strangers – or for some people, with anyone. Indeed, two service users were considered by staff to have 'thrived' in hostels for homeless people that had provided less intensive support than they had thought ideal. Both people had repeated housing difficulties in the past that included unsuccessful stays in supported housing but in the hostel:

> "He seemed to enjoy the camaraderie there with people around him but he didn't have to get too close if he didn't want to."

Workers also mentioned supported housing being a trigger to violence:

> "People perceive him to be quite a high risk because his interactions with other people are often what sparks his behaviour. And yet, at the same time, it's in those environments that you're going to get the intensive support."

Some service users felt frustrated that staff were not helping them to achieve what they wanted: a home of their own. Not getting the accommodation that he wanted may have been a contributory factor in another man leaving the area and almost certainly becoming homeless again. Risk taking and supporting service users to attain the lifestyle they hope for might reduce the risks of disengagement, but there are undoubted difficulties in doing so where someone is perceived as a high risk to others, or where professionals are convinced that the person is unable to manage independent housing. However, even where a service user agreed to go into supported housing, their application could be unsuccessful due to concerns about risk and providers' ability to cherry pick residents:

> "There's such a demand for their housing, you know, they don't have to take people where the challenge is so great. I'm not saying they're deliberately ignoring it – they wouldn't do that. But, given the choice between three and four people where there's an equal need, you know, for that type of housing, obviously the last person they're going to take is someone where the challenge is so high, as it would be with X."

Summary

This chapter provides a wealth of detail about how the service users in this study experienced medication and the difficulties that many had in taking it on a long-term basis. There are no easy solutions here but our hope is that service users' accounts of their experiences will increase professionals' understanding of why some people wish or decide to discontinue taking medication.

While it is well known that use of medication is a contentious issue for mental health services as

well as the law makers, the refusal of some
service users to accept supported housing (often
seen as an essential element of mental health
policy and provision), may be more surprising.
We found that the level of support that service
users wanted and what professionals considered
them to need was an area of potential conflict.

Ultimately, the higher the risk the person is
perceived to pose, the less room they had to
refuse medication and the less likely they were to
be offered independent housing.

7

Conclusion

The study provides an account of service users' perspectives on, and experiences of, posing a former or potential risk to other people. It shows that many service users were deeply distressed about their behaviour when experiencing psychosis and wanted support to reduce the likelihood of them acting in ways that put other people at risk. The study also provides information about the extent of service user involvement in risk assessment and management, as well as care planning, within one mental health trust. The views and perspectives of mental health workers and relatives and friends have also been explored and we highlight many examples of good practice as well as suggest where practice could be more effective.

In the next section we focus on what we think are the key issues arising from the research, and we then pose a series of questions that hopefully service users, relatives, workers, managers and policy makers will find helpful in considering how to achieve valued and effective services.

Being informed about risk

Some service users could not be asked to take part in this research because they did not know that professionals thought them to be a possible risk to other people. In our view, all service users should be informed of such professional opinion. We consider this a civil rights issue. It is also difficult to see how relationships based on trust between professionals and users can develop unless this happens.

Involving service users in risk assessment and management

Service user involvement in risk assessment and management was variable and depended on individual professional initiative. A body of knowledge about how to involve service users considered to pose a potential risk to others in risk assessment and management does not exist. While virtually all professionals said that they discussed concerns with service users – and many professionals were interested in increasing user involvement in their own practice – they did not necessarily use the language of risk and not all service users knew that risk assessment and management was an integral part of the professional role.

A focus on professionally-led approaches to risk assessment and management may also ignore or underplay risks which many service users see as important, such as the disempowering aspects of much mental health provision and the over-emphasis on medication to support individuals experiencing mental distress.

Indeed, the prevailing climate within which mental health workers operate is not helpful towards positive risk taking, defined by Morgan (2000, p 49) as:

> Risk-taking is not negligent abdication of clinical responsibility…. It is about making good quality clinical decisions to support and sustain a course of action that will lead to positive benefits and gains for the individual service user.

We would agree with Morgan that "it is perhaps one of the most difficult concepts to put into practice within a context of a 'blame culture'" (p 49). We also suggest that other factors that impact on its development within practice are the association of mental health problems with dangerousness and the assumption that all risks should be and can be prevented. Professionals are also much less likely to be blamed for unnecessarily restricting service users' lives than for taking positive risks to help them achieve a better quality of life. Professionals and managers need to consider ways in which they can ensure that practice is defensible rather than defensive. Clearly, organisational risk policies and team and organisational culture exert a strong influence on professionals' ability to adopt a positive risk-taking model.

Few professionals were undertaking systematic risk assessment or risk management plans. This is not to say that if they did so, risks would be more accurately assessed or more effectively managed. However, a format for assessing and managing risk could usefully be developed that ensures that service users' views about risks are automatically included.

Professionals in this study were not using actuarial tools such as the MacArthur Risk Assessment Tools, but if they had been, it would have been important to highlight the fact that no risk assessment tool has yet been found that does not have high levels of false positive rates. For example, in research, the MacArthur instrument identified a high-risk group, but 55% of those people did not go on to commit violence (Munro, 2001). Yet the authors suggest that they have a useful tool for clinical practice (Monahan et al, 2000). Indeed, if this or similar tools are used by professionals in practice, it seems to us that service users should know how they are rated and indeed how accurate the measure is.

There is a pressing need for further discussion of these difficult issues, involving both mental health service user groups and professionals.

Holistic focus

Risk assessments should not narrowly focus on mental state and behaviour causing concern but should be a holistic assessment that considers all risks that the person may be experiencing, for example arising from lack of work, poverty, stigma, discrimination or racism, as well as the risks of suicide and self-harm. The continuing

effect of trauma, such as childhood abuse, also needs to be assessed. Risk management plans should address all these concerns.

Discussing risk

A good relationship between the service user and professional within which the service user's qualities were valued was important in discussing risk as were sensitivity and timing, for example to ensure that where a person is experiencing a serious psychotic breakdown such discussion does not cause further distress. Staff concerns about their own safety need to be taken into account, although some of the fears that discussion may lead to violence may be unfounded.

Levels of agreement

The process of negotiation over a care plan that the service user found acceptable and which professionals thought was sufficient to manage the risks they considered to be present could be fraught. Ultimately professionals have the power to decide whether they will accept a person's wishes, for example over where to live or whether to take medication. The study shows varying levels of agreement between service users and professionals about risk and its management. Common ground was more likely where the person's strengths and abilities were valued, where they had a good relationship with a professional that had developed over time and where the support offered was what the person wanted, rather than being imposed.

Involvement in plans made for support

The service users who were articulate and determined had some advantages in that they were able to exert some influence over their care plans, although getting a service that they really wanted was not within their control. Little use was made of advocates for people who found it less easy to express their views.

Information

Accurate information about risk is vital – both to protect others where the person may be a risk and to protect the service user from acting in ways that they would never condone when not experiencing psychosis and which may also lead to restrictions on their liberty. The examples of inaccurate or conflicting information found in the study are a cause for serious concern. We have made many suggestions on how to improve information exchange and accuracy.

Service users were reliant on the professionals working with them in terms of what sort of service they were offered. They were not knowledgeable consumers who knew about the range of services that could be provided to them and a strategy to provide that information is needed.

The following list of questions summarise the good practice examples, suggestions and questions that are dispersed throughout the report and should be read in conjunction with them.

Questions

Assessing and managing risk

- Do service users know that assessing and managing risk is an integral aspect of the role of mental health workers, and do they have written information about this?
- Is there a corresponding focus on service users' strengths and abilities?
- How involved are service users in the assessment of risk both to themselves and to other people? (By involved we do not just mean in a meeting but throughout the whole process of discussing risks, exploring the extent of agreement or disagreement, focusing on what the service user considers important.)
- Are other risks, such as those arising from self harm, abuse, racism, lack of meaningful activity, poverty or discrimination assessed?
- Is there any information that should not be given to service users, that is, scales that assess how high a risk someone is of committing suicide?

- What support needs to be in place for teams and organisations to adopt a positive risk-taking approach?

Information: accuracy, confidentiality and exchange

- Are service users' views sought concerning the accuracy of information held about them?
- Are service users' opinions about any risks included in written documentation and care plans along with a description of the context within which their behaviour occurred?
- Are witnesses sought for serious incidents not agreed between the service user and professional or where there is uncertainty over the level of risk behaviour?
- Is the service user's account also included?
- Do case records have an identifiable section where information about risk can be easily retrieved?
- Do case records have a section, if relevant, containing (1) information from service users about what helps them to stay calm or cool down when agitated or angry and (2) information from staff about successful strategies they have used to achieve the same aim?
- Are information sharing protocols about risk in place for the transmission of information between professionals that include safeguards about confidentiality?
- Are there individual agreements about confidentiality negotiated between service users, professionals and relatives or friends, if involved?
- Is professional opinion about risk properly substantiated and is there information about context and the chronology of any incidents?

Issues related to people from black or minority ethnic groups

- Are service users who are subject to racial abuse or attack offered the choice of discussing this with a member of staff from a black or minority ethnic group (or an appropriate black or minority ethnic organisation)?
- Do investigations of black or minority ethnic patients attacked while hospital in-patients

always consider whether such attacks are racially motivated?

- Are interpreters trained about confidentiality and the requirement to relay *exactly* what service users say? Are they given some basic training in mental health issues?

Care planning

- How involved are service users in drawing up care plans and how much real influence do they have over them?
- How much preparation and support for service users as well as flexibility over size of care plan meeting is there?
- Are service users able to use advance directives and are they informed about advocacy services?
- Do all service users have written relapse plans?
- Do services evaluate service users' views about the professionals involved in their lives and offer them a change of worker if required?
- Are long-term service users offered appointments with the same doctor rather than trainee doctors who change every six months?
- How can a service user's wish to maintain a care plan be respected when the worker with whom the plan was developed leaves?
- How much negotiation is there between service user and professional over type and dosage of medication?
- How systematically are service users monitored for side-effects?
- How much is the desire to get a service user settled in supported housing fulfilling their needs or those of professionals for them to be somewhere 'safe'?

Information

- Are service uses given written information about (1) the full range of services available within mental health services, the voluntary sector and self-help groups and (2) what mental health policy says should be in place within local services?
- Do service users receive information about the side-effects of medication?

Relatives

- Do relatives have information about how to access help or support for service users?
- Are protocols in place to ensure a coordinated response within community services to relatives' or friends' requests for assistance?
- Are relatives or friends given written relapse plans where the service user agrees this?

References

Appleby, L. (2001) *Safety first: Five year report of the National Confidential Inquiry into suicide and homicide by people with mental illness*, London: DoH.

Appleby, L., Shaw, J. and Amos, T. (2000) 'Sudden unexplained death in psychiatric in-patients', *British Journal of Psychiatry*, vol 176, pp 405-06.

Boardman, J., Grove, J., Perkins, R. and Shepherd, G. (2003) 'Work and employment for people with psychiatric disabilities', *British Journal of Psychiatry*, vol 182, pp 467-8.

Browne, D.A. (1997) *Black people and sectioning: The black experience of detention under the civil sections of the Mental Health Act*, London: Little Rock Publishing.

Campbell, P. and Lindow, V. (1997) *Changing practice: Mental health nursing and user empowerment*, London: Royal College of Nursing and MIND.

DoH (Department of Health) (1990) *The care programme approach for people with a mental illness referred to the specialist psychiatric services*, HC (90) 23, London: DoH.

DoH (1994) *NHS Executive guidance on the discharge of mentally ill people and their continuing care in the community*, HSG (94) 27/LASSl (94) 4, London: DoH.

DoH (1999a) *Effective care co-ordination in mental health services: Modernising the care programme approach*, 16736 HSD, London: DoH.

DoH (1999b) *Reform of the Mental Health Act 1983: Proposals for consultation*, Cm4480, London: DoH.

DoH (2000) *Reforming the Mental Health Act*, London: DoH.

DoH (2002a) *Draft Mental Health Bill*, Cm 5538-1, London: DoH.

DoH (2002b) *Mental health policy implementation guide: Dual diagnosis good practice guide*, London: DoH.

Emerson, R.M. and Pollner, M. (1975) 'Dirty work designations: their features and consequences in a psychiatric setting', *Social Problems*, vol 23, pp 243-54.

Estroff, S.E. and Zimmer, C. (1994) 'Social networks, social support, and violence among persons with severe, persistent mental illness', in J. Monahan and H.J. Steadman (eds) *Violence and mental disorder: Developments in risk assessment*, Chicago, IL: University of Chicago Press.

Faulkner, A. and Layzell, S. (2000) *Strategies for living: A report of user-led research into people's strategies for living with mental distress*, London: The Mental Health Foundation.

Fernando, S. (ed) (1995) *Mental health in a multi-ethnic society: A multi-disciplinary handbook*, London: Routledge.

Fernando, S., Dnegwa, D. and Wilson, M. (1998) *Forensic psychiatry, race and culture*, London: Routledge.

Grounds, A. (1995) 'Risk assessment and management in clinical context', in J. Crichton (ed) *Psychiatric patient violence: Risk and response*, London: Gerald Duckworth & Co.

Harris, E.C. and Barraclough, B. (1997) 'Suicide as an outcome for mental disorder: A meta-analysis', *British Journal of Psychiatry*, vol 170, pp 205-28.

Health Select Committee (2000) *Provision of NHS mental health services (fourth report)*, London: The Stationery Office (www.parliament.the-stationery-office.co.uk/pa/cm199900/cmselect/cmhealth/3).

Hetherington, R., Baistow, K., Katz, I., Mesie, J. and Trowell, J. (2002) *The welfare of children with mentally ill parents: Learning from inter-country comparisons*, Chichester: Wiley.

Isacsson, G. and Rich, C.L. (2001) Management of patients who deliberately harm themselves, *British Medical Journal*, vol 322, pp 213-15.

Keating, F., Robertson, D., McCulloch, A. and Francis, E. (2002) *Breaking the circles of fear*, London: Sainsbury Centre for Mental Health.

Kinderman, P. (2000) *Recent advances in understanding mental illness and psychotic experience*, London: British Psychological Society (also available at: www.bps.org.uk/docdownload/docdownload3.cfm?category_ID=19&document_ID=159).

LAC (Local Authority Circular) (96)8 (1996) *Guidance on supervised discharge (after-care under supervision) and related provisions*, London: DoH.

Langan, J. (1999) 'Assessing risk in mental health', in P. Parsloe (ed) *Risk assessment in social care and social work*, London: Jessica Kingsley Publishers.

Langan, J. and Lindow, V. (2000) 'Risk and listening', *Openmind no 101*, January/February, pp 14-15.

MacArthur Research Network on Mental Health and the Law (2001) *The MacArthur violence risk assessment study: Executive summary* (available at http://macarthur.virginia.edu/risk.html).

Monahan, J., Steadman, H.J., Robbins, P.C., Silver, E., Appelbaum, P.S., Grisso, T., Mulvey, E.P. and Roth, H.R. (2000) 'Developing a clinically useful actuarial tool for assessing violence risk', *British Journal of Psychiatry*, vol 176, pp 312-19.

Morgan, S. (1999) *Clinical risk management: A clinical tool and practitioner manual*, London: The Sainsbury Centre for Mental Health.

Morgan, S. (2000) *Clinical risk management: A clinical tool and practitioner manual*, London: Sainsbury Centre for Mental Health.

Munro, E. (2001) Book review of Blumenthal, S. and Lavender, T. (2000) *Violence and mental disorder: A critical aid to the assessment and management of risk*, Journal of Forensic Psychiatry, vol 12, no 1, pp 248-54.

Munro, E. (2004, in proof) 'A simpler way to understand the results of risk assessment instruments', *Children and Youth Service Review*, vol 26.

Munro, E. and Rumgay, J. (2000) 'Role of risk assessment in reducing homicides by people with mental illness', *British Journal of Psychiatry*, vol 176, pp 116-20.

National Assembly for Wales (2001) *Adult mental health services for Wales: Equity, empowerment, effectiveness, efficiency: Strategy document*, Cardiff: National Assembly for Wales.

Parker, C. and McCulloch, A. (1999) *Key issues from homicide inquiries: An analysis carried out by MIND*, London: MIND.

Petch, E. (2001) 'Risk management in the UK mental health services: An overvalued idea?', *British Journal of Psychiatry*, vol 25, pp 203-05.

Robinson, A. (1997) *Reach for the moon*, Sidmouth: Freedom Press.

Sayce, L. (1995) 'Response to violence: A framework for fair treatment', in J. Crichton (ed) *Psychiatric patient violence*, London: Duckworth.

Scottish Executive (2000) *Risk management*, Report of the Mental Health Reference Group, Edinburgh: Scottish Executive.

Stanley, N. and Manthorpe, J. (2001) 'Reading mental health inquiries: messages for social work', *Journal of Social Work*, vol 1, no 1, pp 77-99.

Steadman, H., Mulvey, E.P., Monahan, J., Robbins, P.C., Applebaum, P.S. and Grisso, T. (1998) 'Violence by people discharged from acute inpatient facilities and by others in the same neighbourhoods', *Archives of General Psychiatry*, vol 55, no 5, pp 393-401.

Taylor, P.J. and Gunn, J. (1999) 'Homicides by people with mental illness: myth and reality', *British Journal of Psychiatry*, vol 174, pp 9-14.

Thornicroft, G. (2000) *Shaping the new Mental Health Act: Key messages from the Department of Health research programme: supervision and coercion studies* (available at www.doh.gov.uk/mhar/mha_use3.htm).

Warner, R. (1994) *Recovery from schizophrenia: Psychiatry and political economy*, London: Routledge.

Wilson, M. and Francis, J. (1997) *Raised voices: African-Caribbean and African users' views of mental health services in England and Wales*, London: MIND.

Appendix: The methodology

Location of research

The service users came from one urban area in England and were in-patients in two hospitals within the same mental health trust which we have called Middletown Hospital and Valley Hospital. Middletown Hospital is a traditional mental hospital, set in the country and serving a wide area, including the inner-city of the area. The mental health facilities of Valley Hospital are newly built wards in the grounds of a general hospital serving other parts of the same urban area, as well as rural areas not included in the research. Both hospitals were served by the same social services department. The urban area was commonly seen as having underfunded mental health services, although assertive outreach teams were being established as the research took place.

Timescale

The project started in October 1998 and was agreed by the research ethics committees of the two Trusts in May 1999. The two Trusts merged in April 1999 with two senior management reorganisations subsequently taking place. These reorganisations involved us in informing different sets of people about our research in order to gain their cooperation and slowed down the process of gaining consents from service users.

We gained our first referrals in July 1999 and had to pursue consultant psychiatrists and remind them of the study in order to gain referrals.

Finding the sample

As is common in much mental health research, we had no direct contact with service users until they had agreed to take part in the research. We saw this as good practice and it was also required by the two ethics committees that gave us permission to conduct the research. We sent our checklist form to consultant psychiatrists and asked them to nominate people who fulfilled the selection criteria. Once this was done, we were given the name of the person's keyworker and their unique NHS patient number. We then sent this person an information leaflet and consent form about the research for the patient. We also provided an information leaflet for the keyworker. Since initially we only had the hospital number until the service user agreed to meet us, the process of gaining agreement was often protracted. For example, if patient numbers were not known by ward staff, they had to contact the medical records office to find out who the patient was.

The plan was to interview 20 service users across the two hospitals as well as staff and relatives or friends where the service user agreed to this. When we had meetings with key staff to gain their agreement for the research to take place, they were confident that these numbers would pose no problem. However, it proved extremely difficult to find enough people to make up this number. There may be several reasons for this. Some people were not informed that professionals considered them to pose a potential risk to other people. Also, while some consultant psychiatrists nominated several people, others needed many reminders. We do not mean to be too critical here since there were several consultant posts vacant during the research period, which clearly contributed to this situation. However, it does underline the difficulty of gaining contact to service users.

The service users

After a long and protracted process, we interviewed 17 services users (15 men and 2 women) whose contact with psychiatric services varied from nearly 40 years to less than a year. Interviews took place around the time of their discharge from hospital. Six months later, we re-interviewed 14 service users (12 men and 2 women). Three service users were not interviewed at Phase 2. Despite repeated attempts it proved impossible to make contact with one service user in person and another service user let us know via his keyworker that he did not want to be interviewed. Both men were from minority ethnic backgrounds. The third service user, who was white, had chosen to lose contact with services.

Another two people had agreed to be interviewed but one was discharged and had not been allocated a keyworker through whom we could make contact. The keyworker for another person said that any contact with us would unsettle the service user. Although we suggested contact a few months later, the keyworker did not agree to this.

Another 32 people suggested to us were not interviewed, for reasons given in Table 1.

The majority of those not interviewed were white men. For comparison purposes, we had hoped to select equal numbers of men and women and also to select sufficient numbers of people from minority ethnic groups. However, this was not possible, given the number of consents that we received. The age and ethnic background (self-defined) of the 17 service users interviewed are given in Tables 2 and 3.

Service users from minority ethnic groups were given the choice of being interviewed by a researcher from a minority ethnic group and two took up this option.

Service user agreement to interview others associated in their care

We made it clear to service users that interviews with other people about their situation was optional. With one exception, service users agreed that we could interview mental health professionals. The person who withheld consent disagreed with the need for treatment and with professional views about his situation. Four service users also chose not to nominate a relative or friend to be interviewed. At Phase 1 the interviews with professionals included the ward nurse, whereas at Phase 2 a ward nurse was only interviewed where service users had been readmitted to hospital.

Table 1: Reasons for not being interviewed

Reason	Number
Agreed but then refused	3
Refused	14
Consent could not be obtained before cut-off point	7
Discharged before contact made and lost to services	3
Discharged before contact made and not allocated keyworker in the community who could inform them of the study	1
Checklist form filled in but not considered a risk by keyworker[a]	4
Total	32

Note: [a] For example, a woman who hit a ward nurse but who was otherwise not considered a risk to others.

Table 2: Age

Age	Number
Under 20	1
20-29	7
30-39	5
40-49	3
50-59	1

Table 3: Ethnic background

Ethnic background	Number
Asian/White UK mixed parentage	1
Black African	1
Black British	1
South Asian	1
White UK	13

Relatives and friends who took part

Thirteen of the 17 service users we met nominated at least one relative or friend that we could interview, making a total of 20 interviews with 10 relatives (4 mothers, 1 father, 1 stepfather, 2 sisters, 2 brothers) and 6 friends over the two interview phases. Some relatives/ friends were interviewed once, while others were interviewed at both interview phases. One service user nominated both parents who were each interviewed twice.

Mental health staff

With one exception, all service users nominated several members of staff at each interview phase. One service user gave permission for only one member of staff at each phase to be interviewed and one of those did not agree to be interviewed. This service user did not think that other workers would give a fair picture of him. A few service users did not want us to meet a particular category of staff, such as psychiatrists or ward staff.

We carried out 78 interviews with 56 members of staff nominated by the service user. The number of interviews per staff member varied from six (interviewed about three service users at both interview phases) to once (interviewed about one service user at one interview phase only). In only two instances was the same doctor interviewed at both phases. Ward nurses were only interviewed at Phase 1 unless the person was an in-patient again at the second interview. The types of staff interviewed, by gender, are shown in Table 4.

Fifty-four of the 56 staff interviewed were white, the majority of whom were British. The remaining two staff were Black African and Asian respectively. While length of time since qualification varied across the professionals, overall this was an experienced workforce.

Refusals

One relative did not wish to be interviewed and four workers refused – two on the basis of being too busy, one because they had had little involvement with the service user and another because of concerns about the impact on their relationship with the service user.

Table 4: Types of staff interviewed, by gender

Type of staff	Female	Male	Total
Ward nurses			
Registered mental health nurses	9	5	14
Student nurse	0	1	1
Doctors			
Consultant psychiatrists	2	9	11
Non-consultant psychiatrists	1	0	1
Senior House Officers (SHO)	4	0	4
Social workers	6	2	8
Community Psychiatric Nurses (CPN)	1	5	6
Housing workers	1	2	3
Day service staff	1	4	5
Community specialist staff[a]	1	2	3
Total	26	30	56

Note: [a] Clinical psychology or occupational therapy.